PICTURE BOOK OF
NORTH AMERICAN BUTTERFLIES

I0756612

"It flies with beautiful wings and joins the earth to heaven. It drinks only nectar from the flowers and carries the seeds of love from one flower to another. Without butterflies, the world would soon have few flowers."

— Trina Paulus

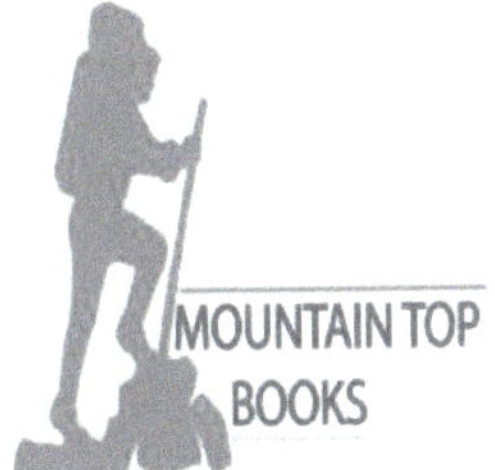

Copyright © 2020 Mountain Top Books
www.amazon.com/author/mountaintopbooks
All Rights Reserved.

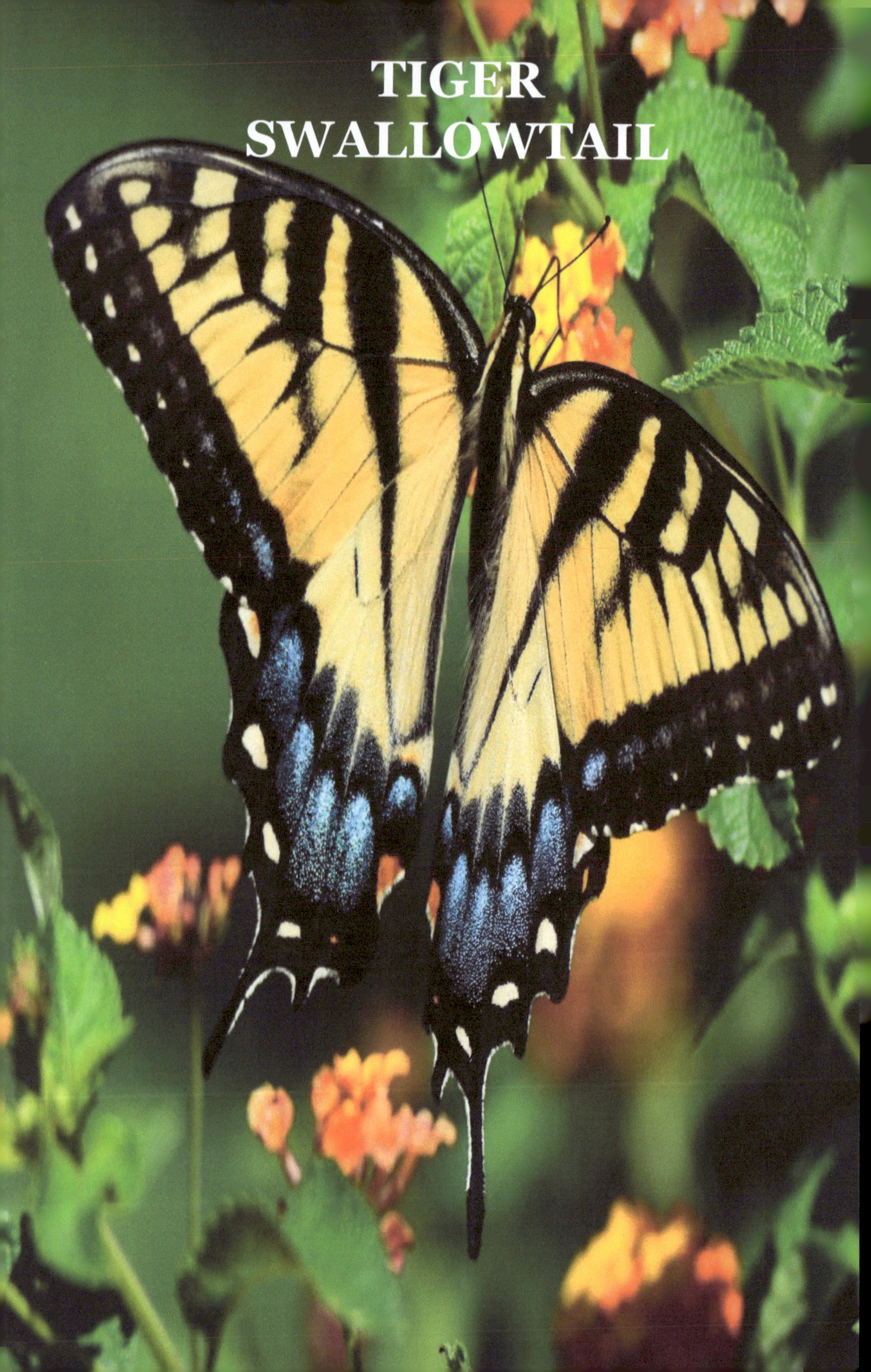

TIGER
SWALLOWTAIL

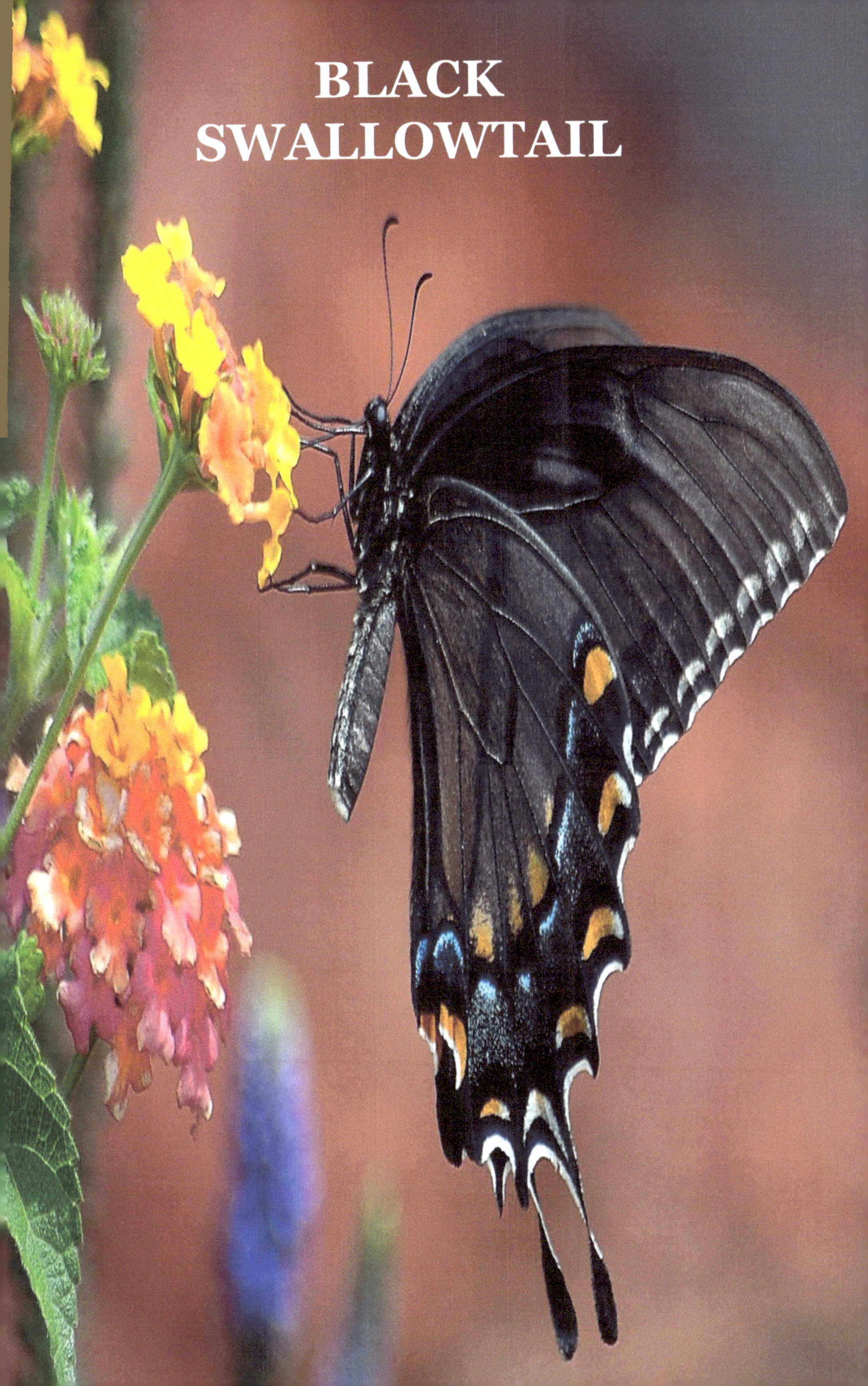
BLACK
SWALLOWTAIL

PAPILIO MACHAON

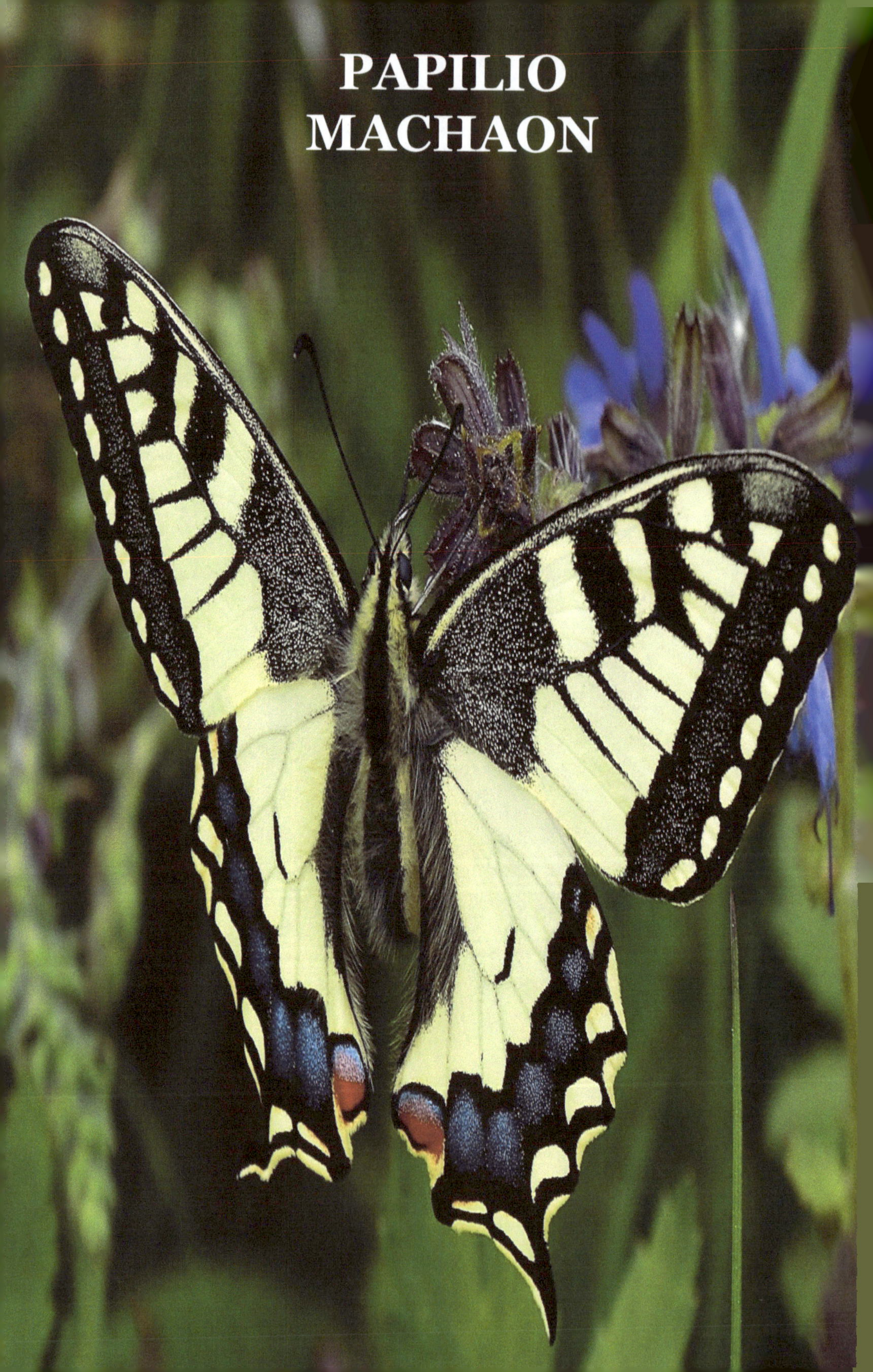

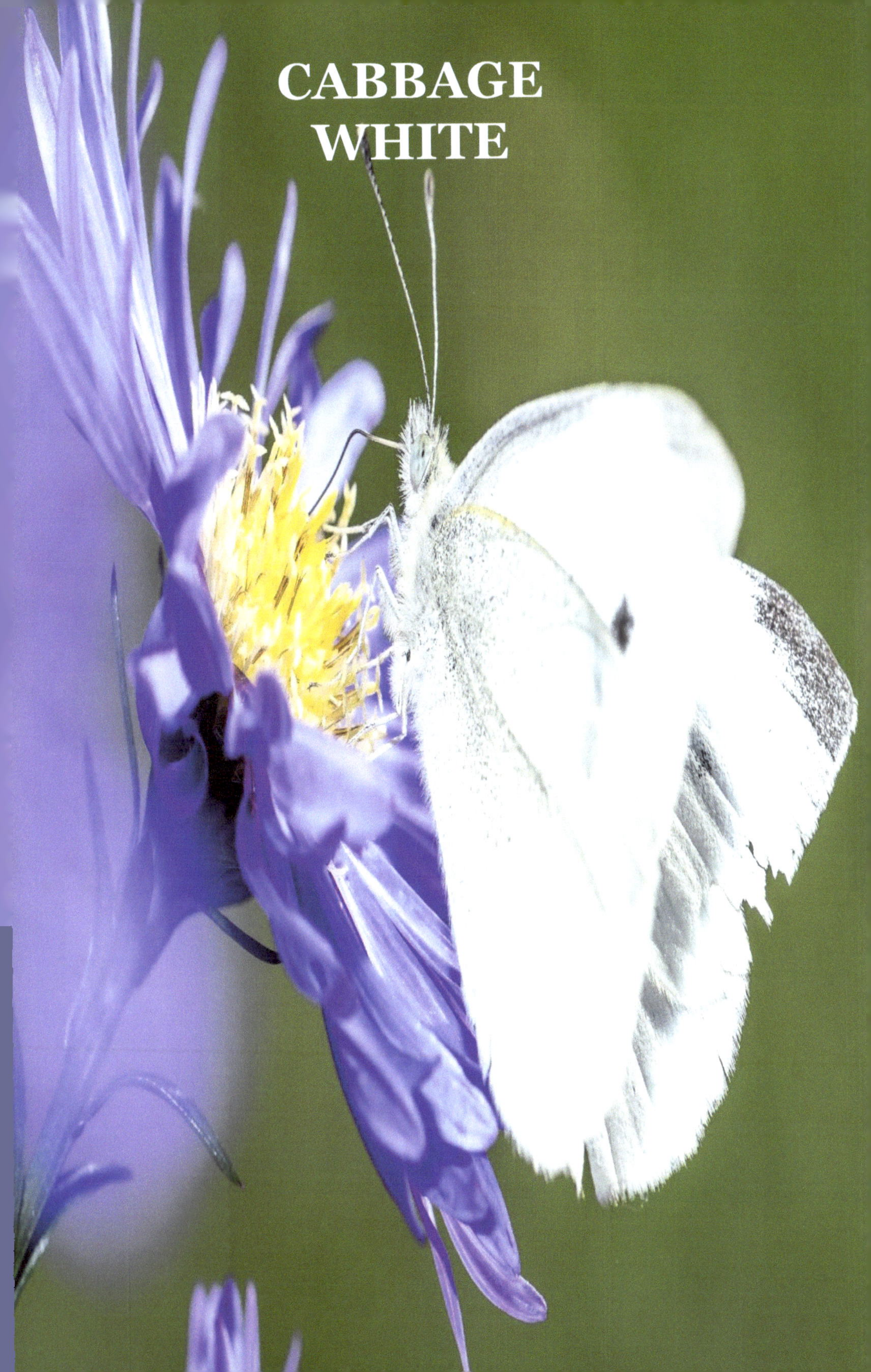

CABBAGE
WHITE

SPRING AZURE

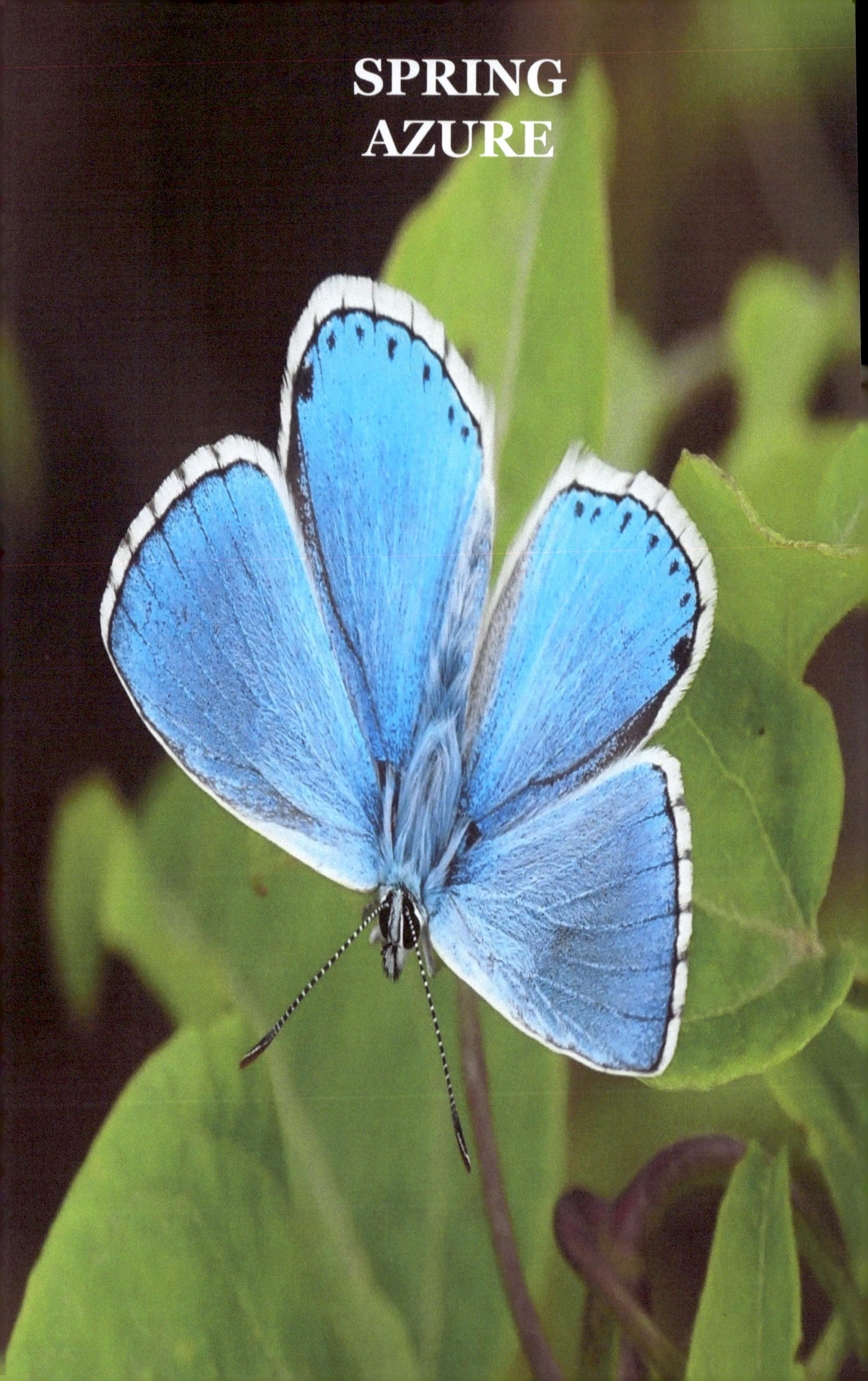

SUMMER AZURE

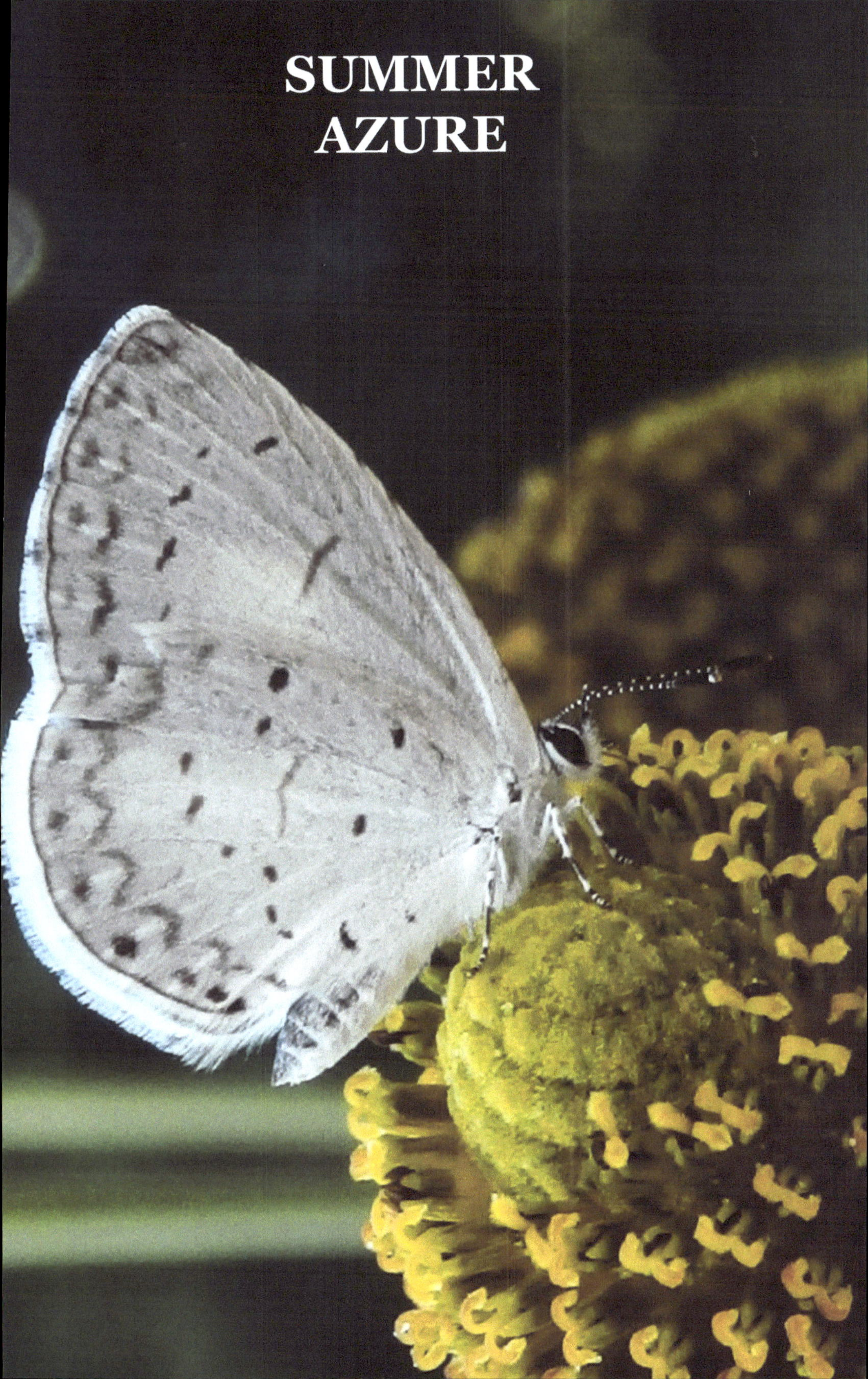

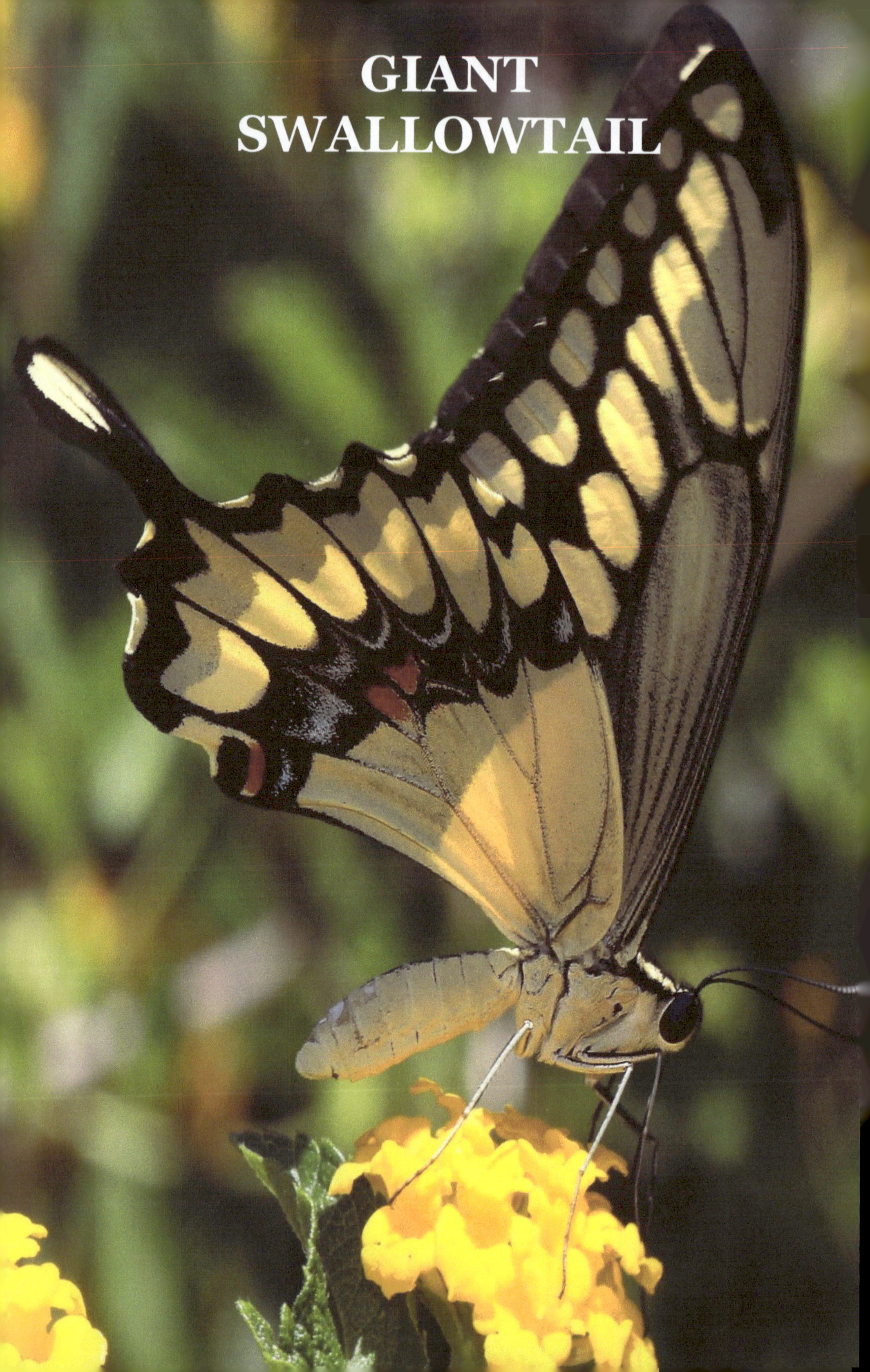
GIANT
SWALLOWTAIL

MONARCH

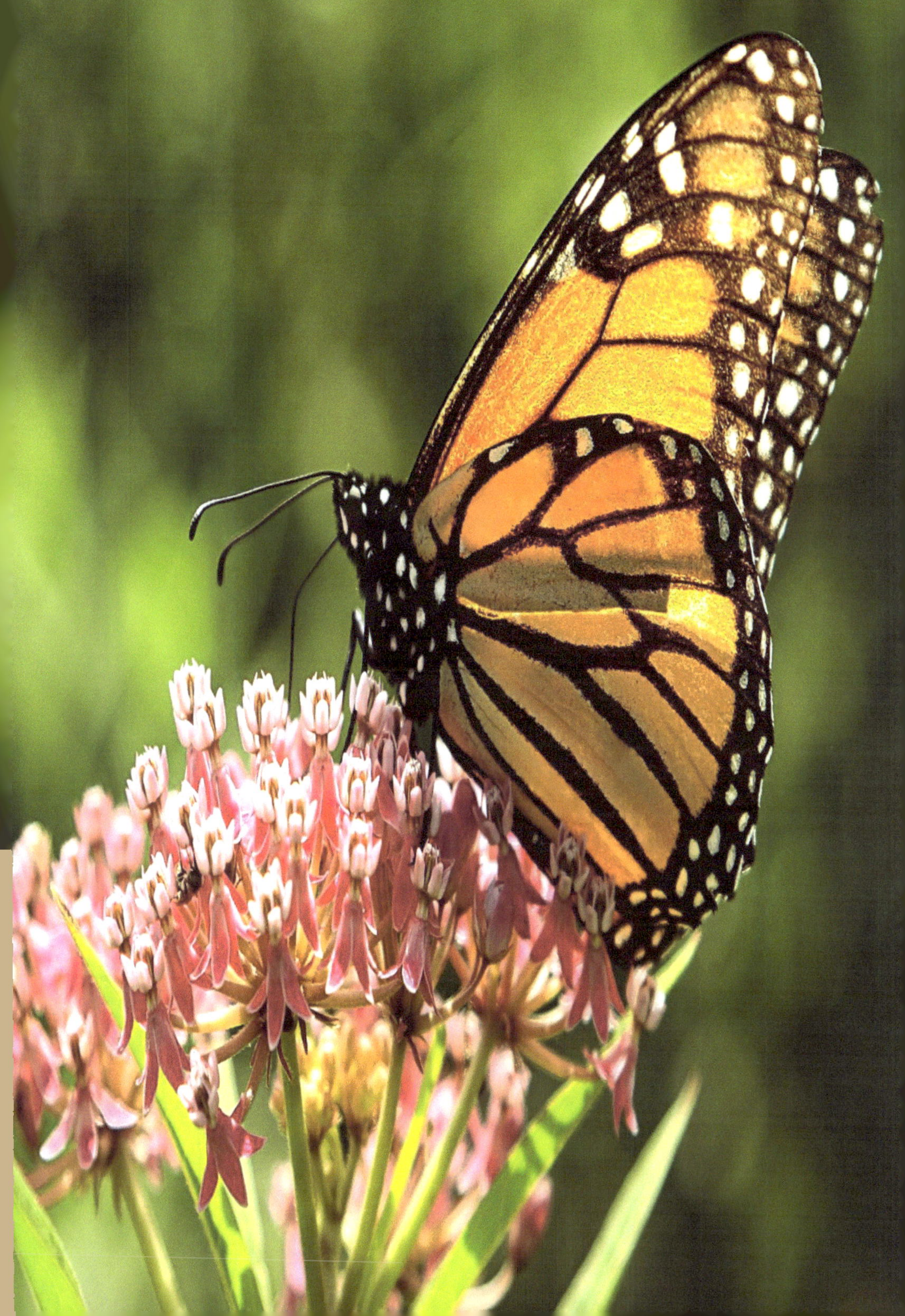

VICEROY

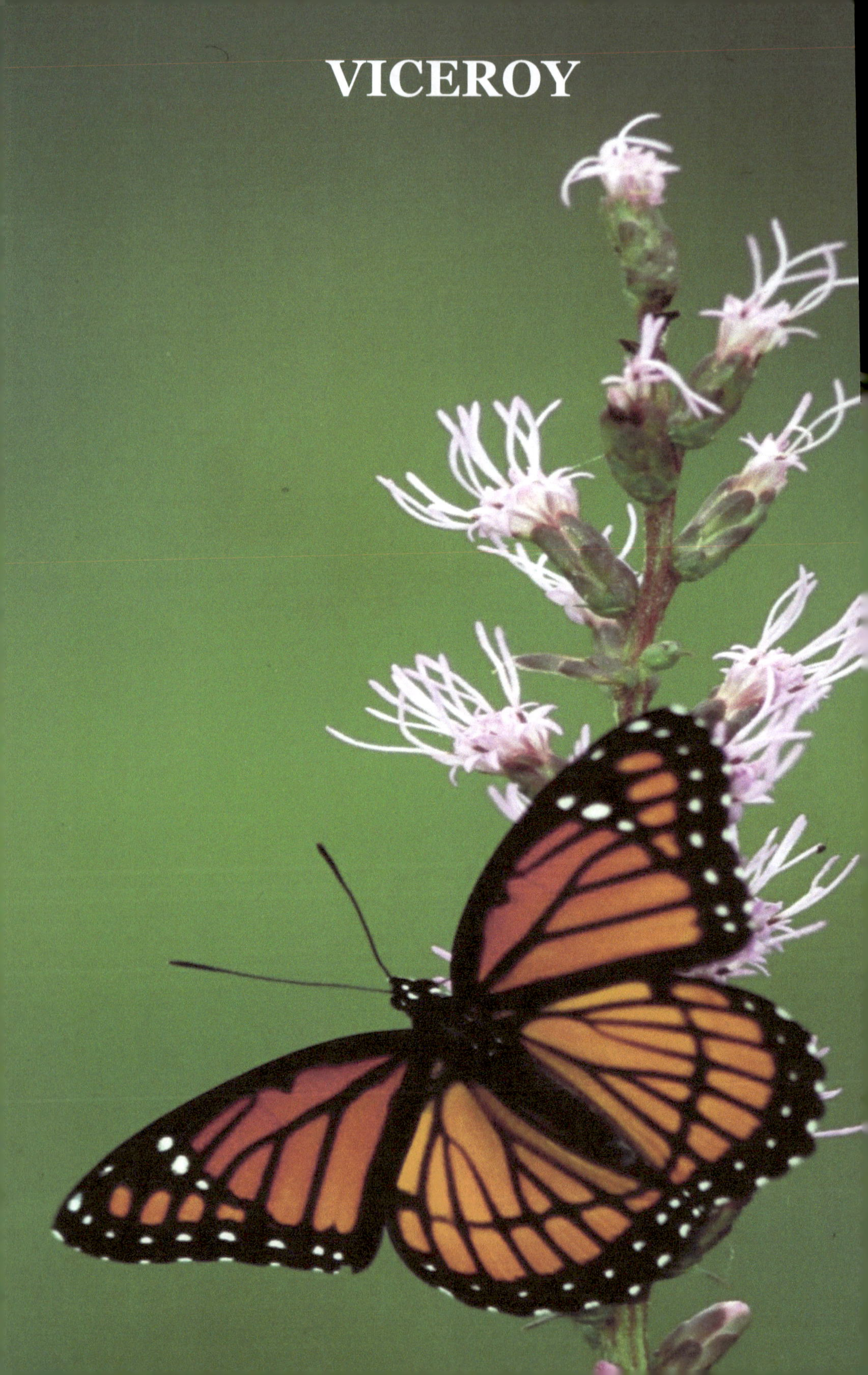

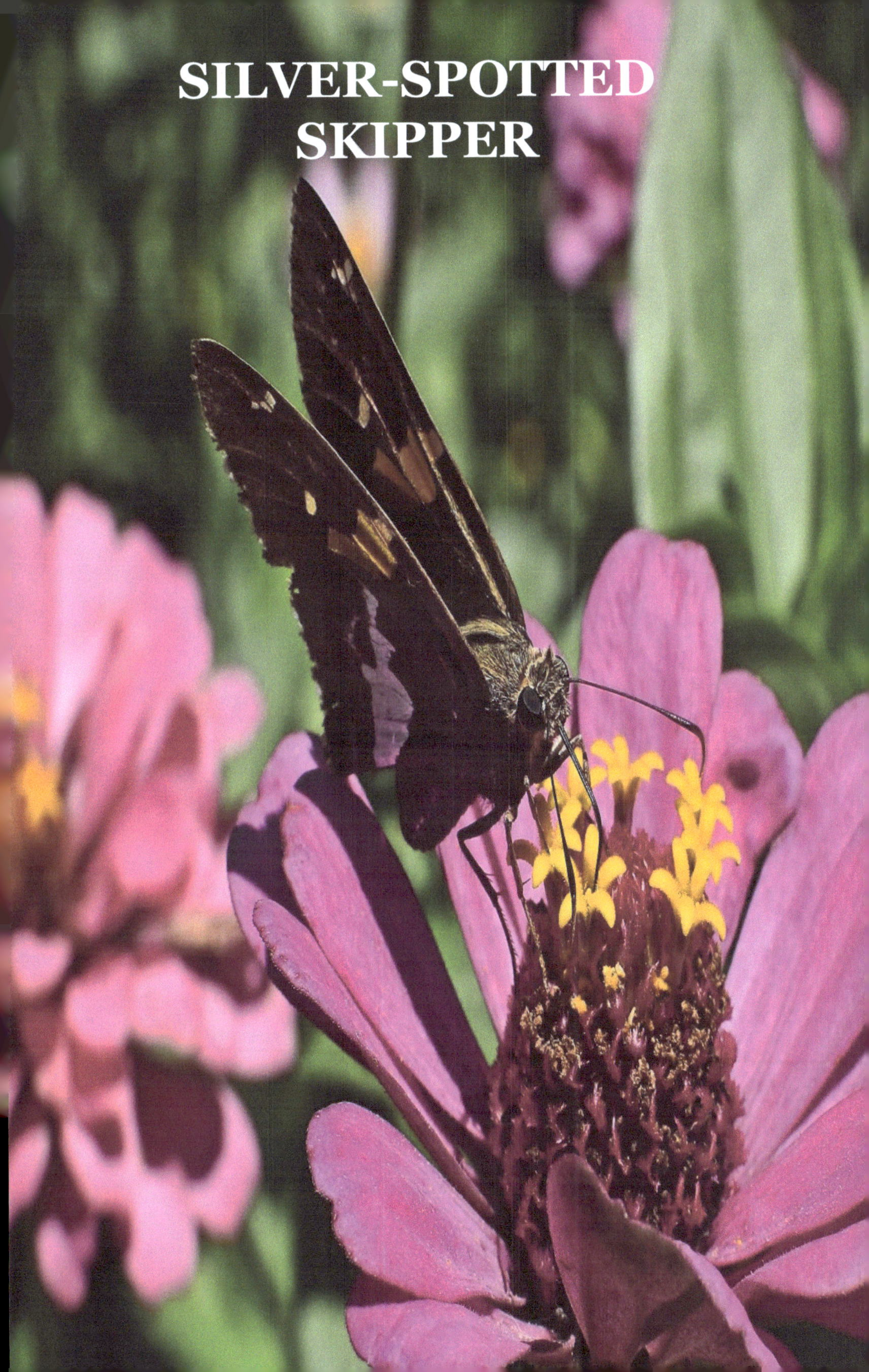
SILVER-SPOTTED
SKIPPER

MALACHITE

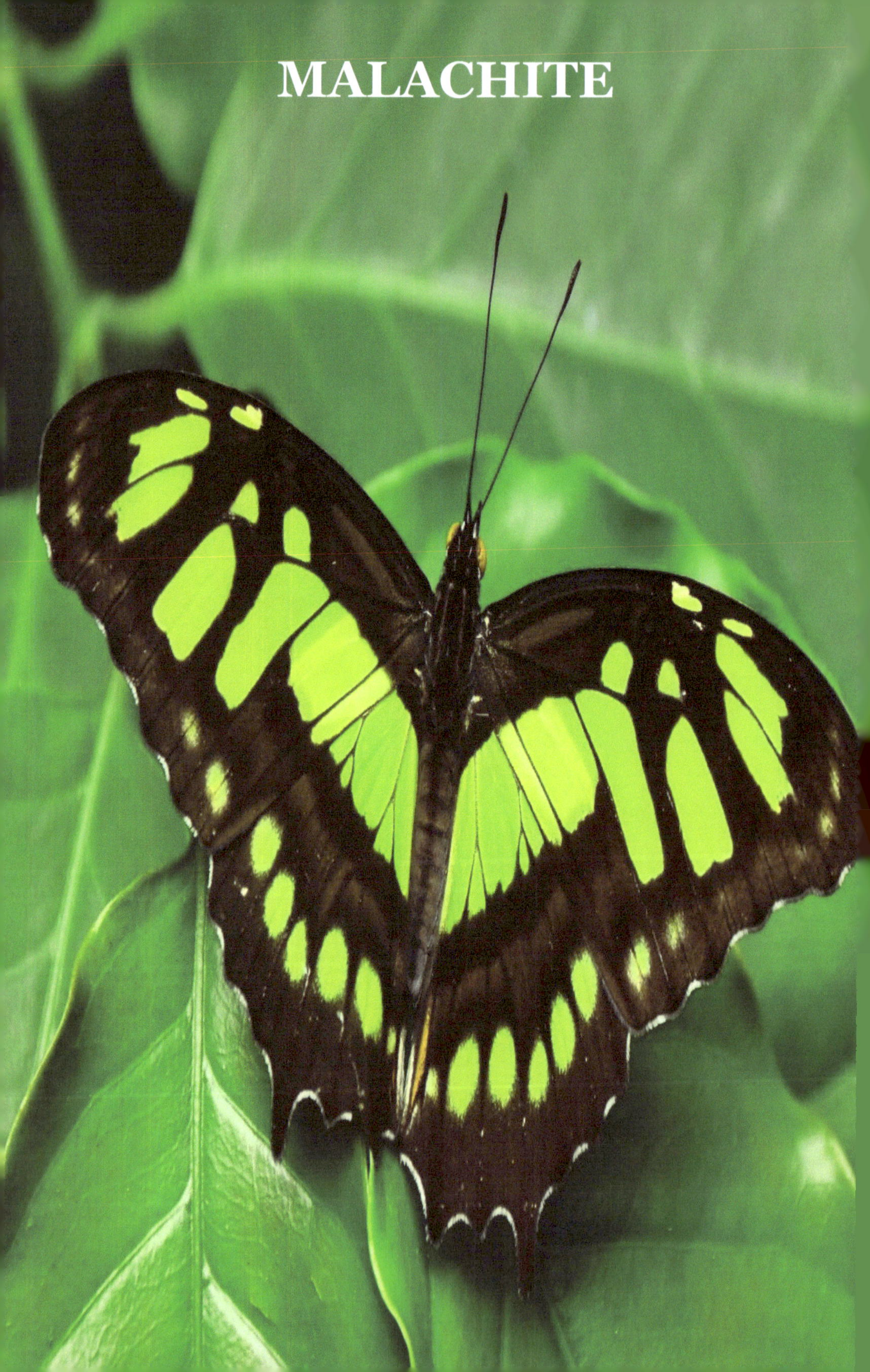

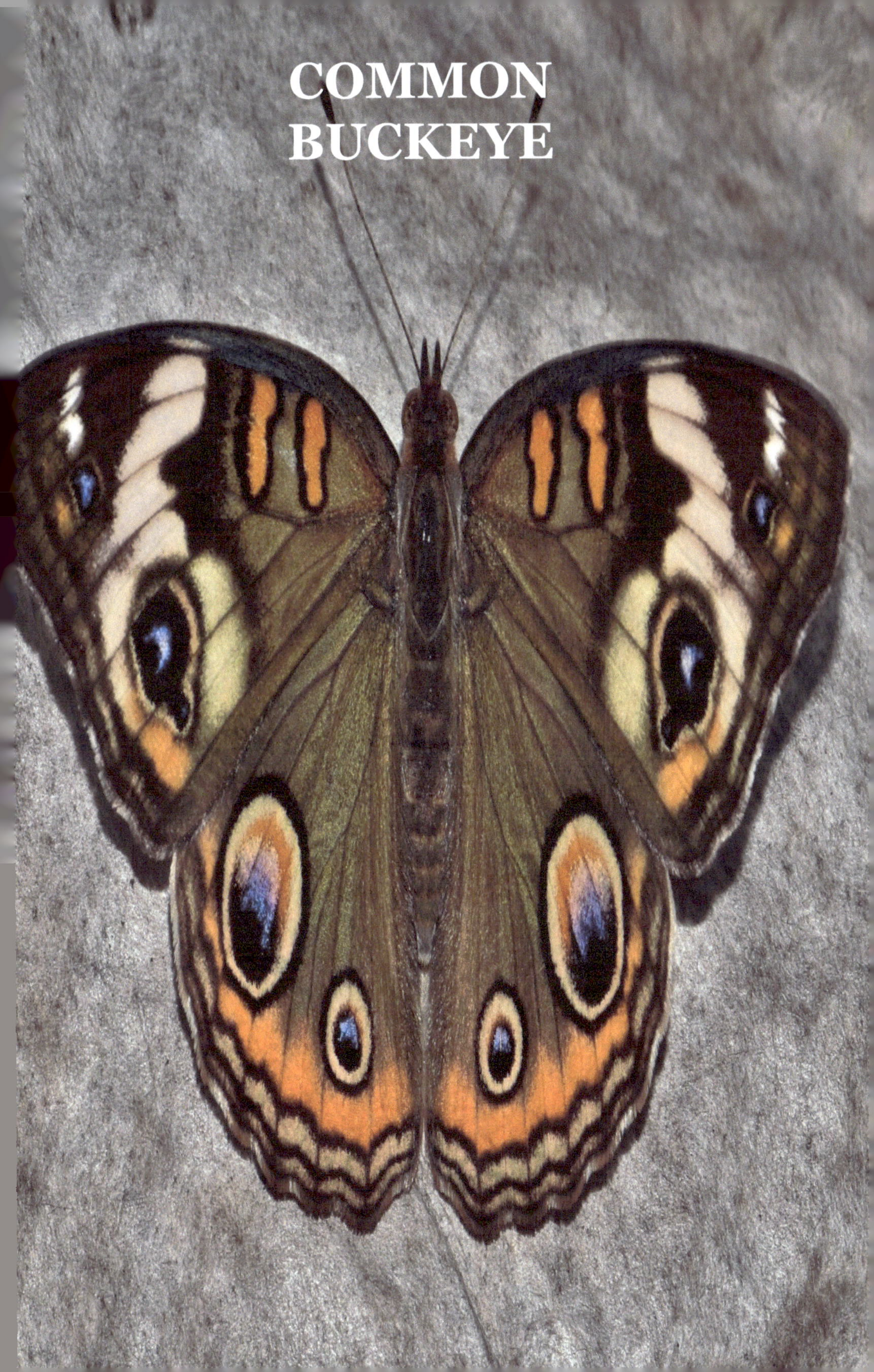
COMMON
BUCKEYE

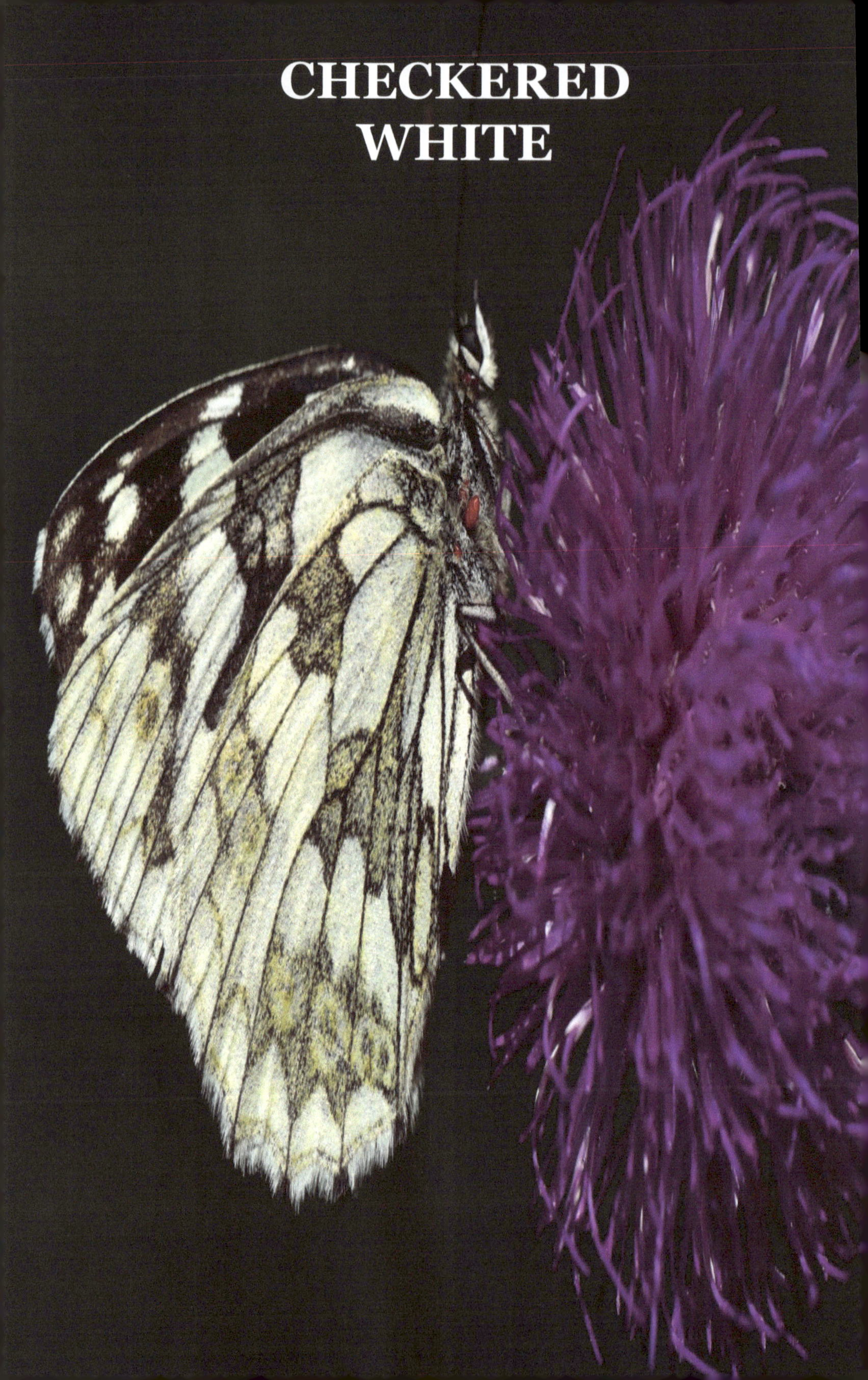

CHECKERED
WHITE

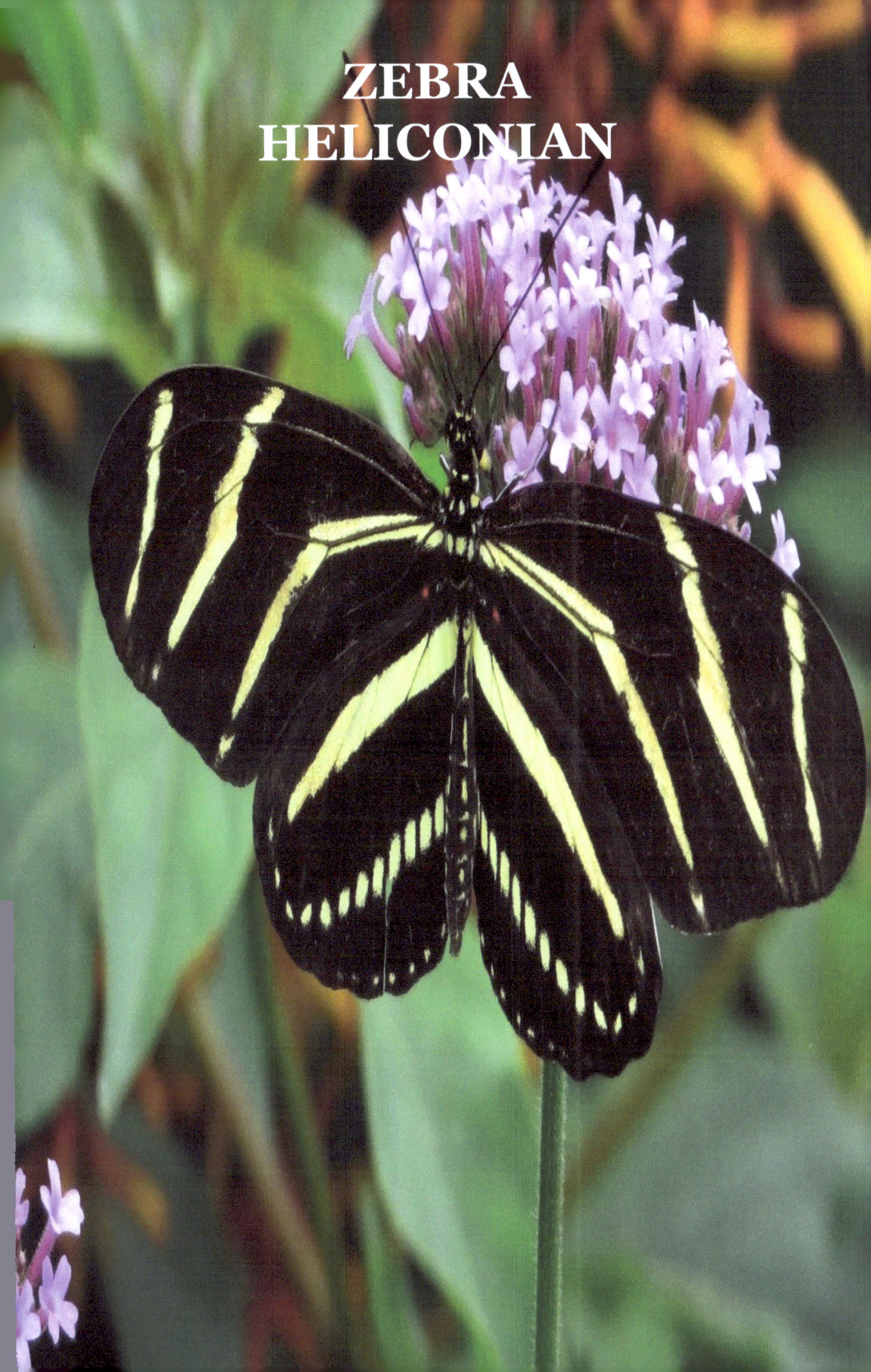ZEBRA
HELICONIAN

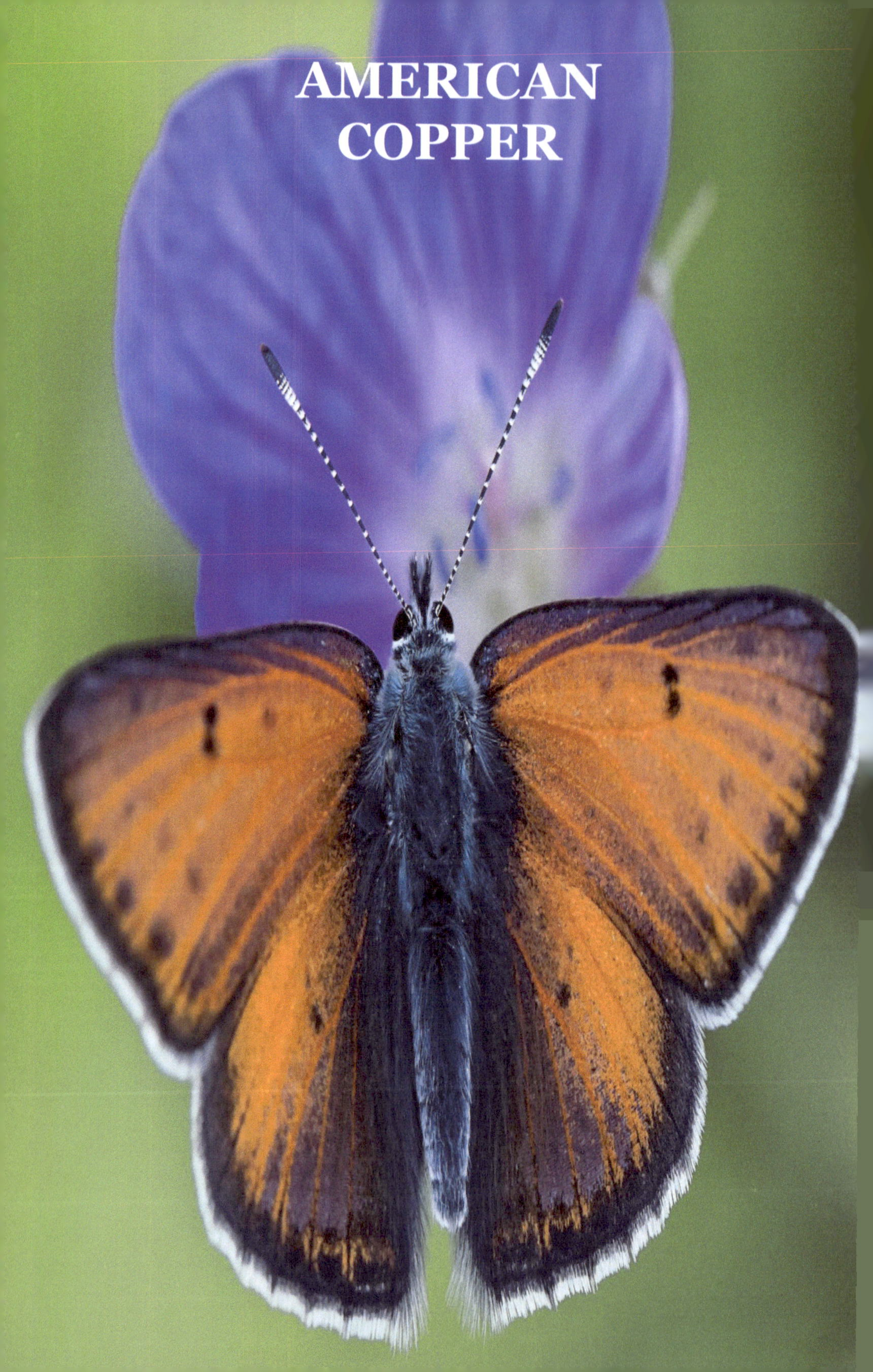
AMERICAN
COPPER

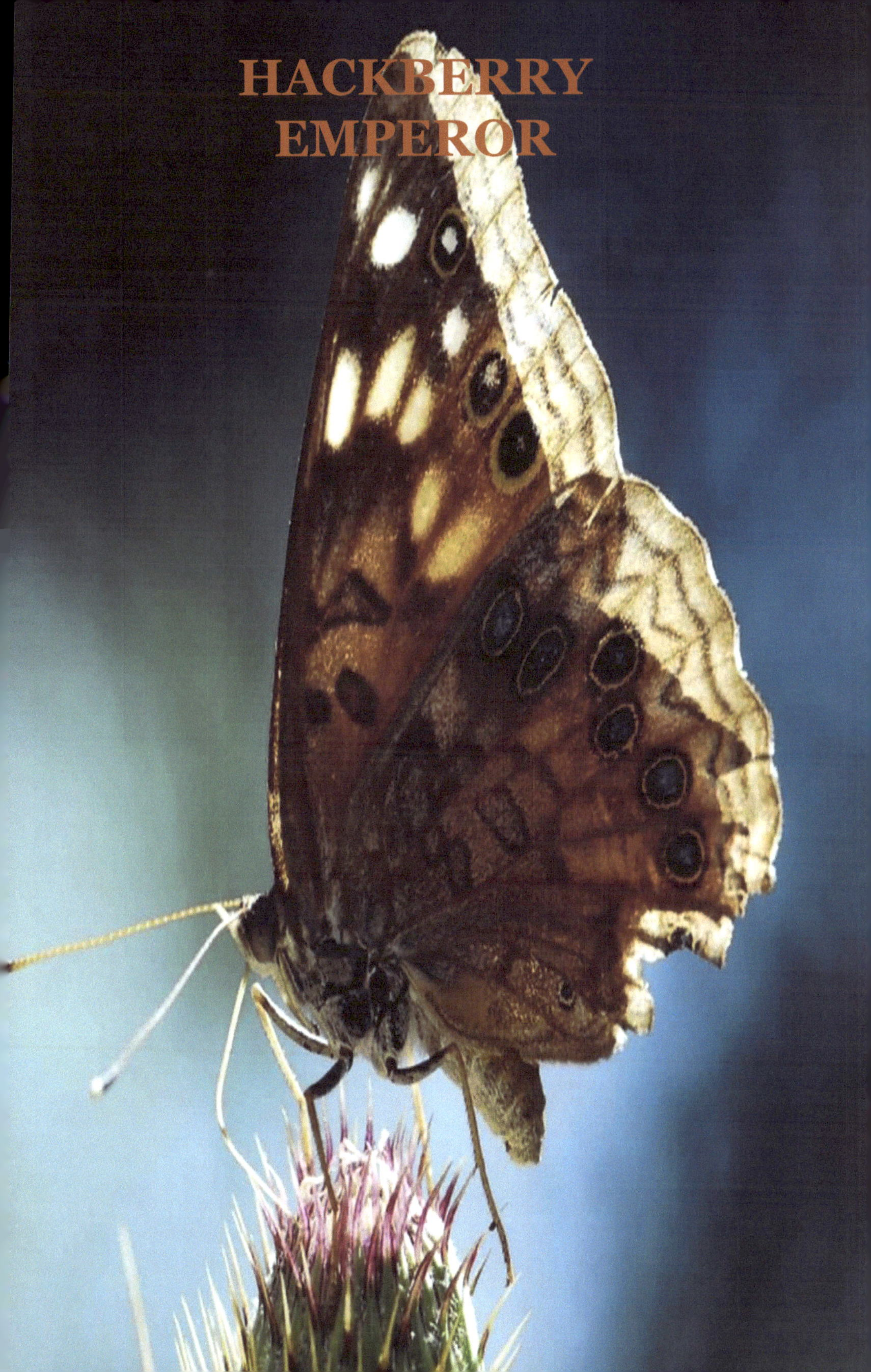
HACKBERRY
EMPEROR

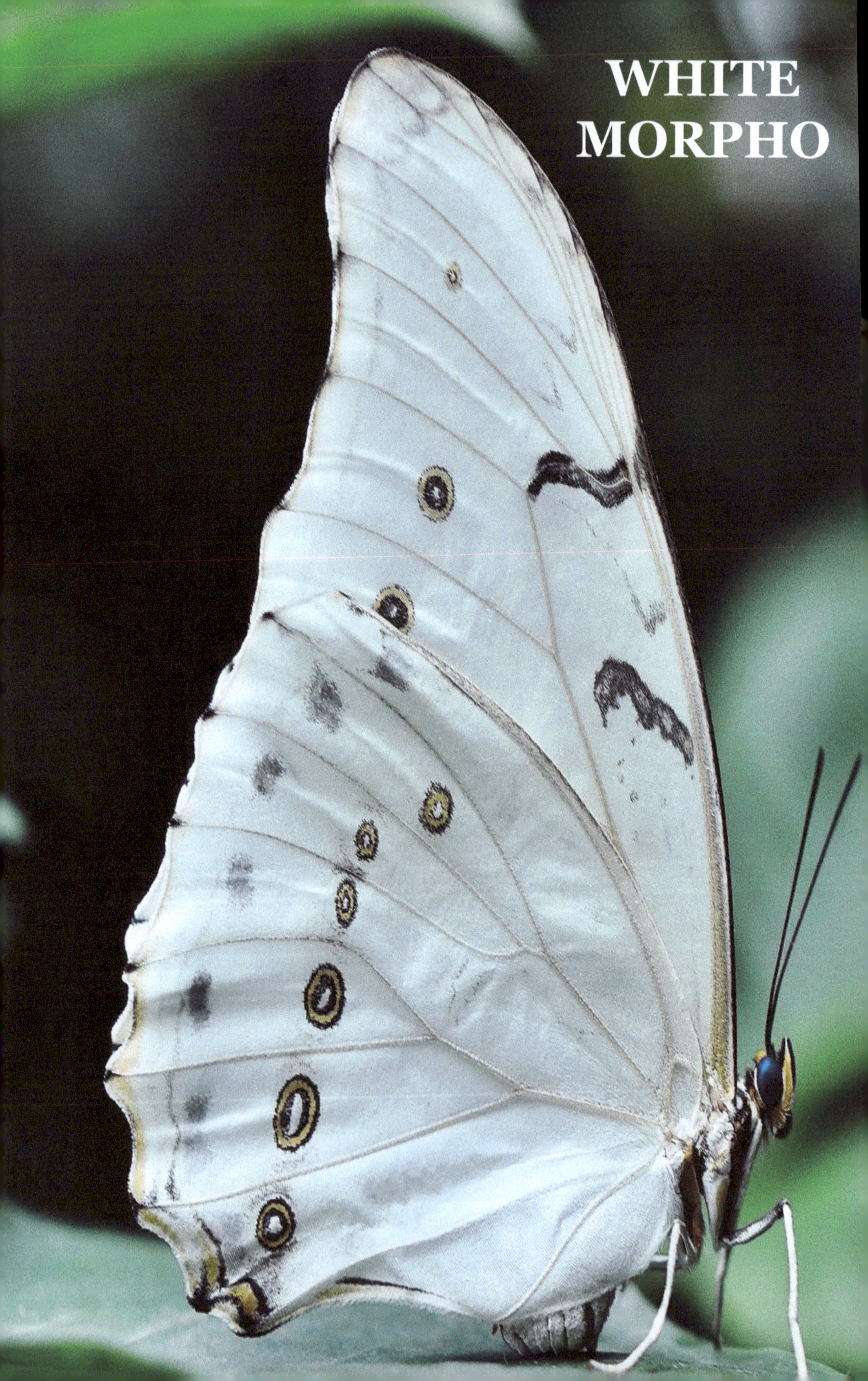
WHITE
MORPHO

RINGLET

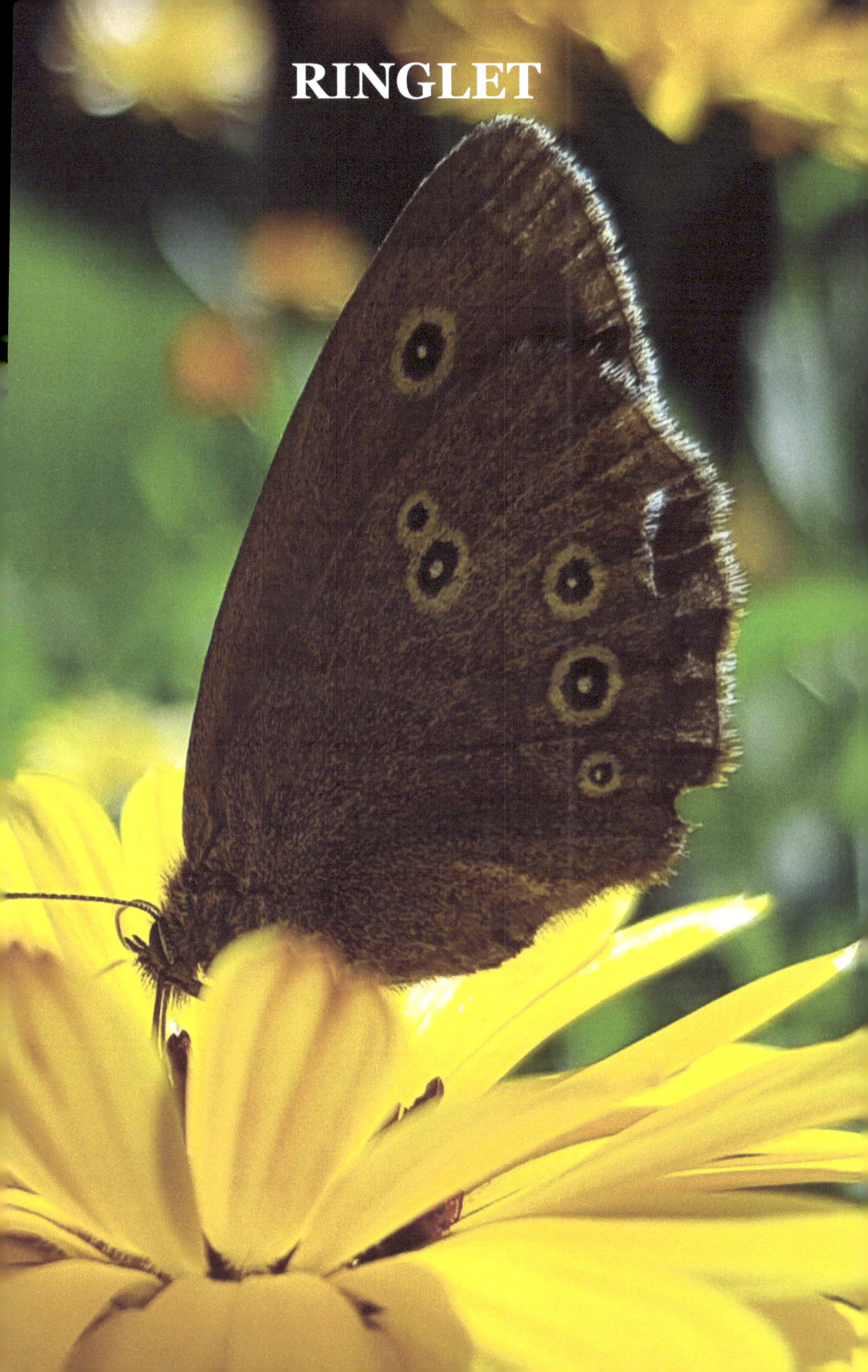

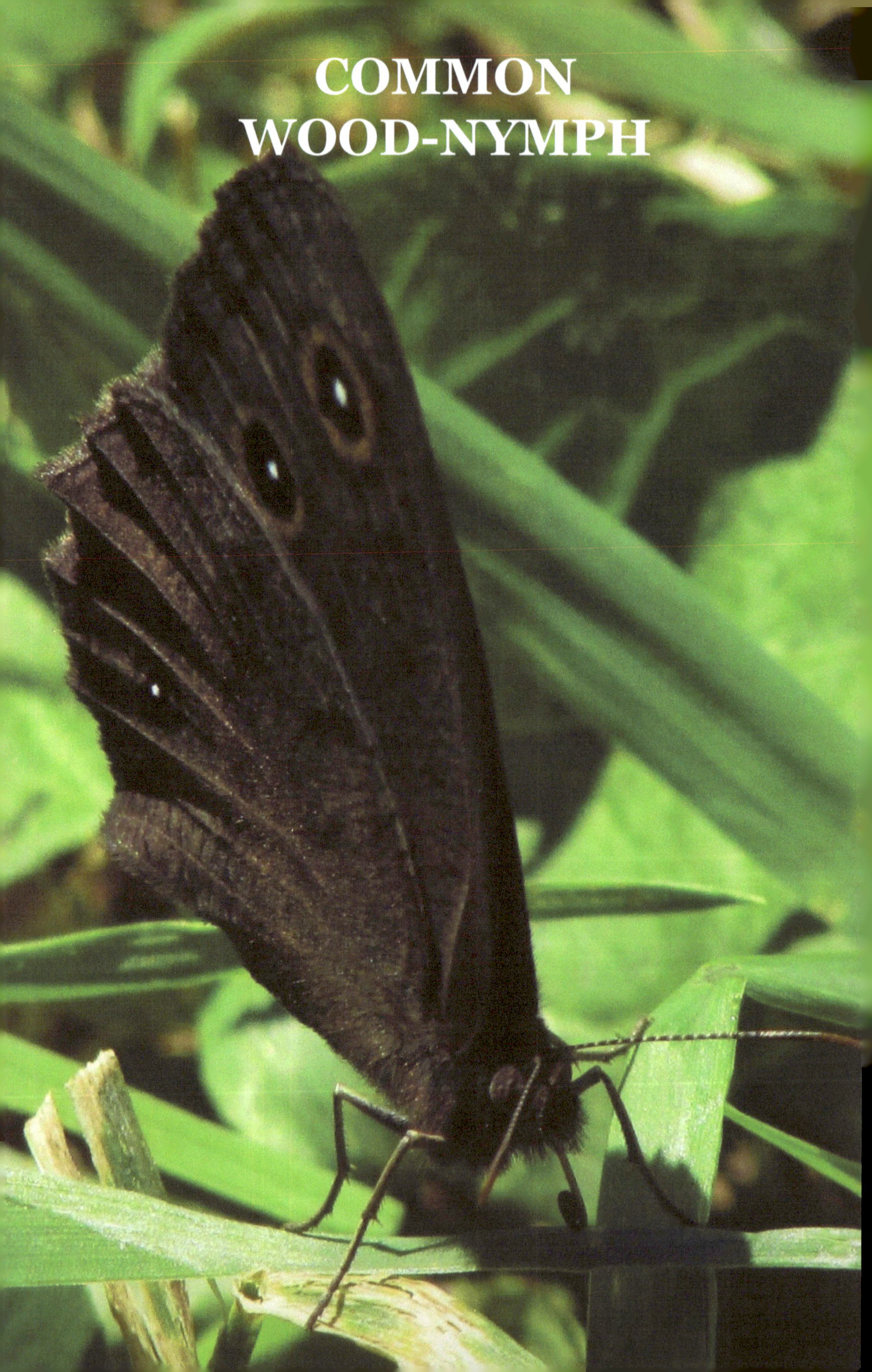

COMMON
WOOD-NYMPH

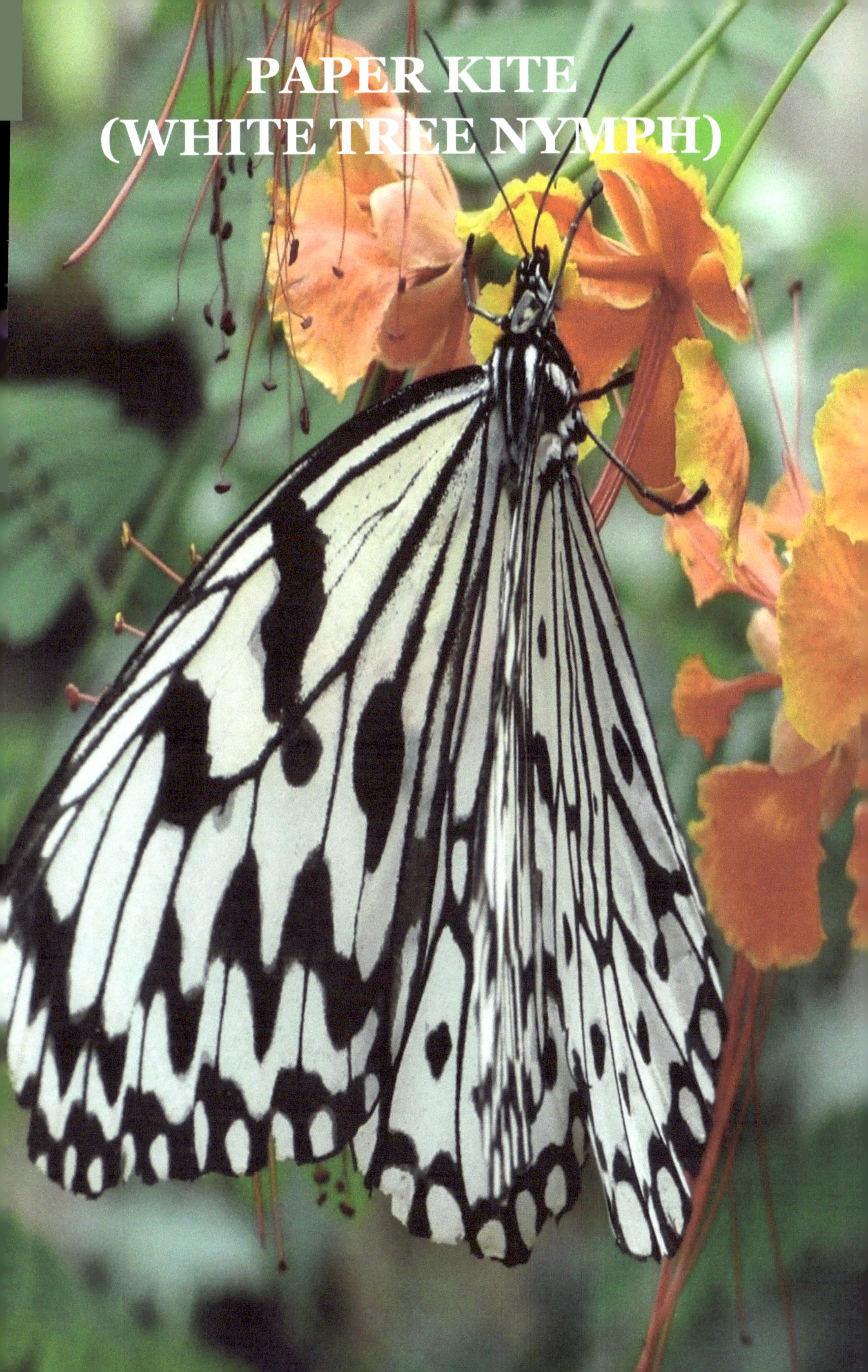

PAPER KITE
(WHITE TREE NYMPH)

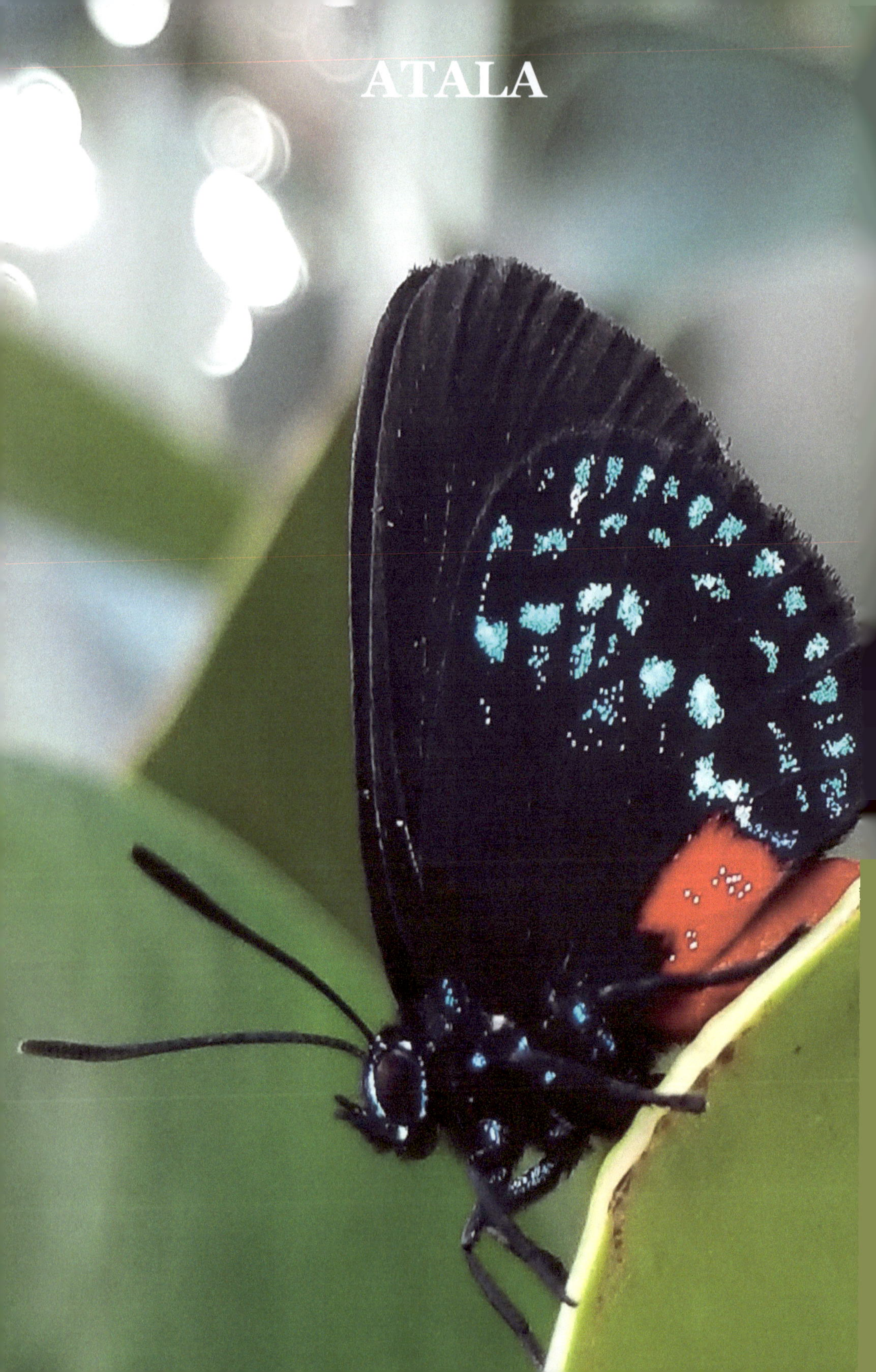

ATALA

POSTMAN

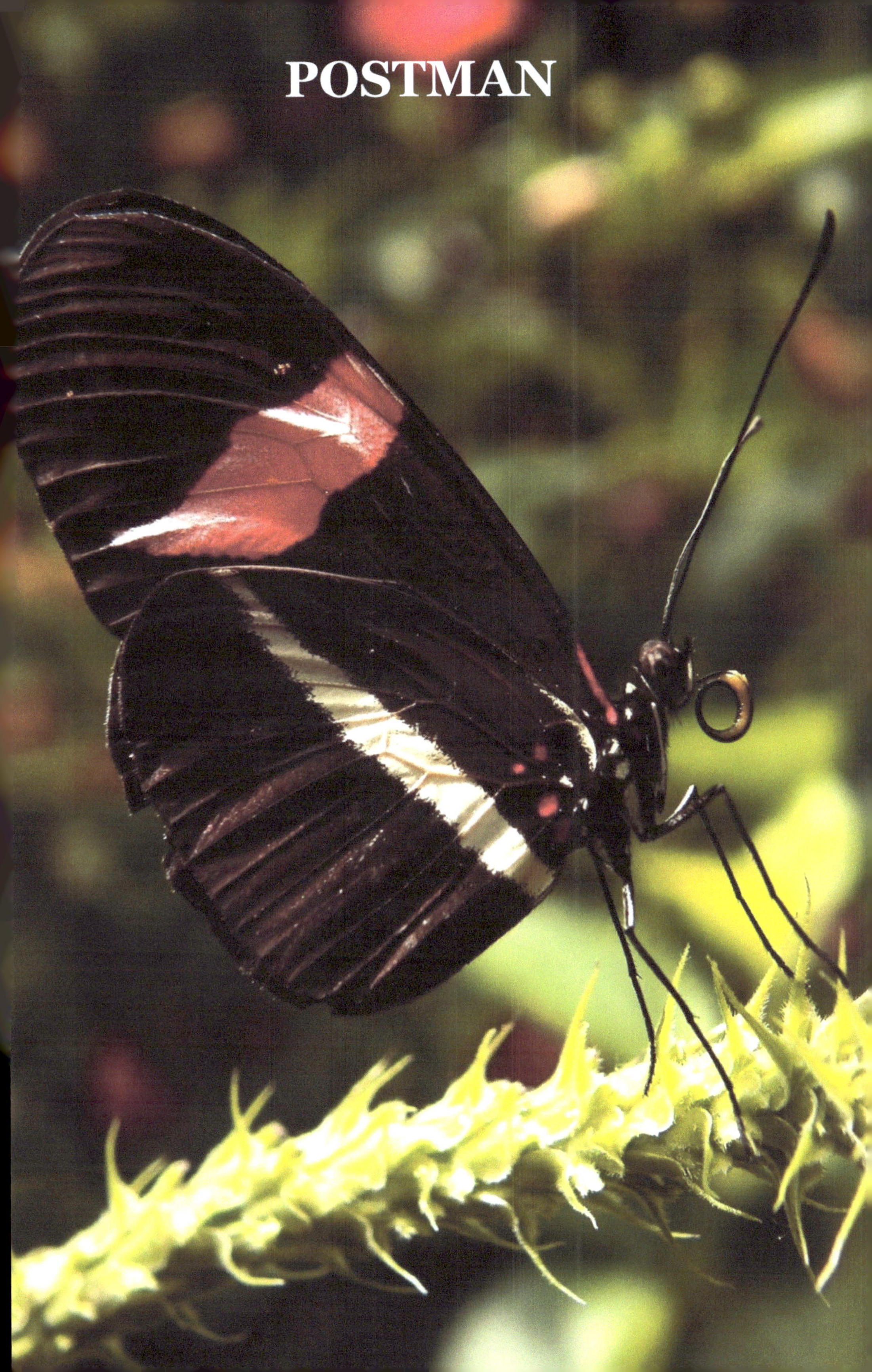

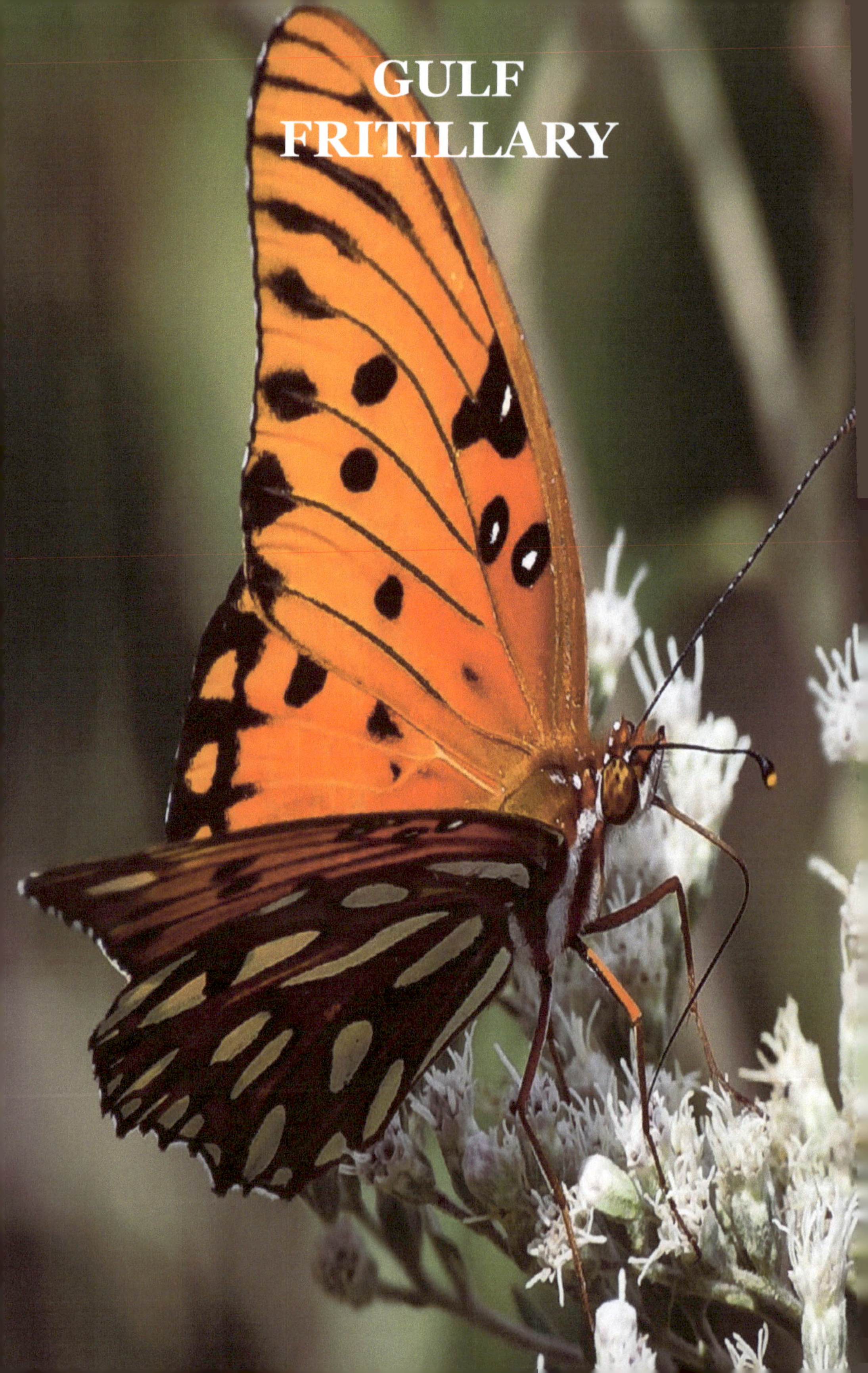

GULF
FRITILLARY

QUEEN

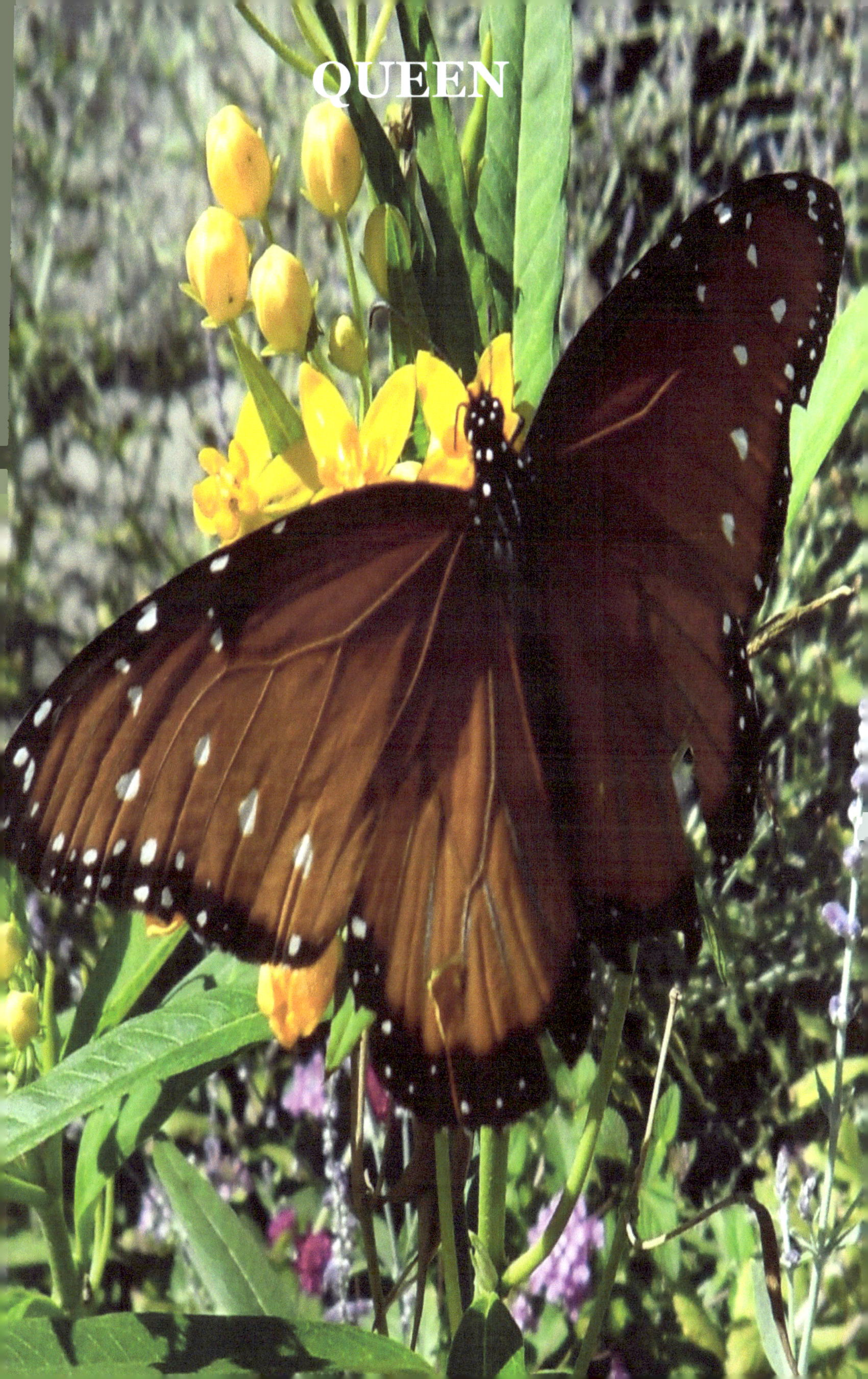

VARIEGATED FRITILLARY

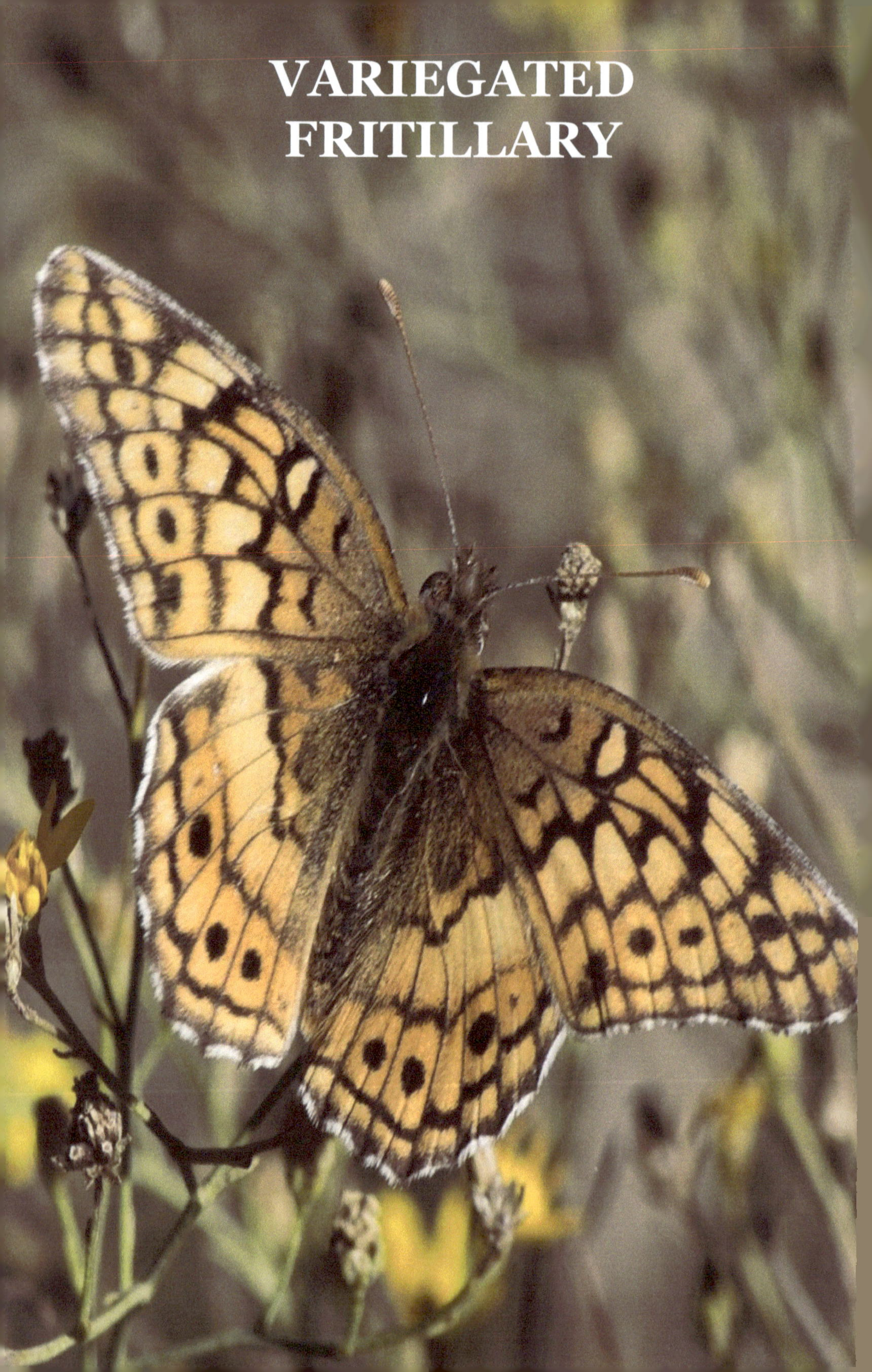

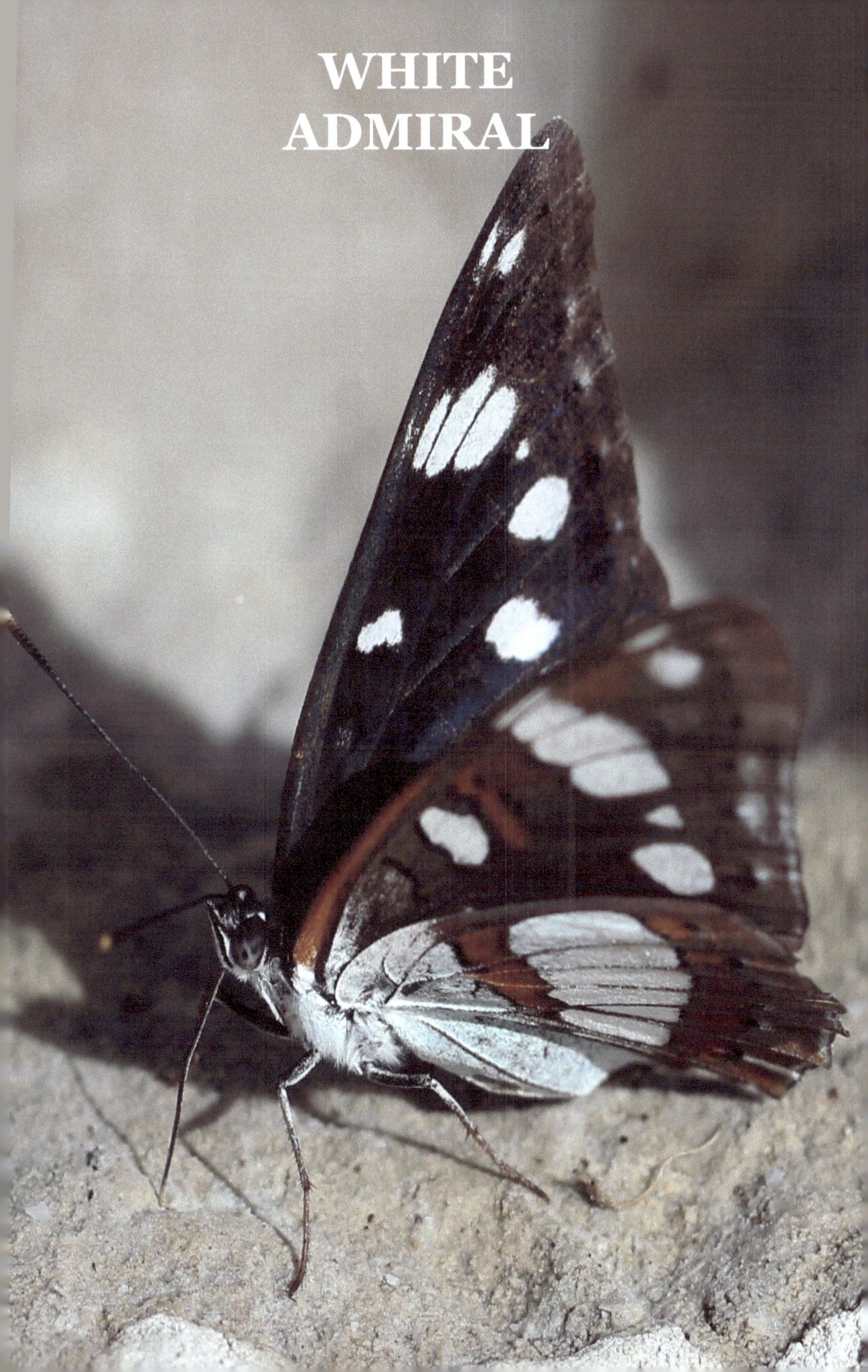
WHITE
ADMIRAL

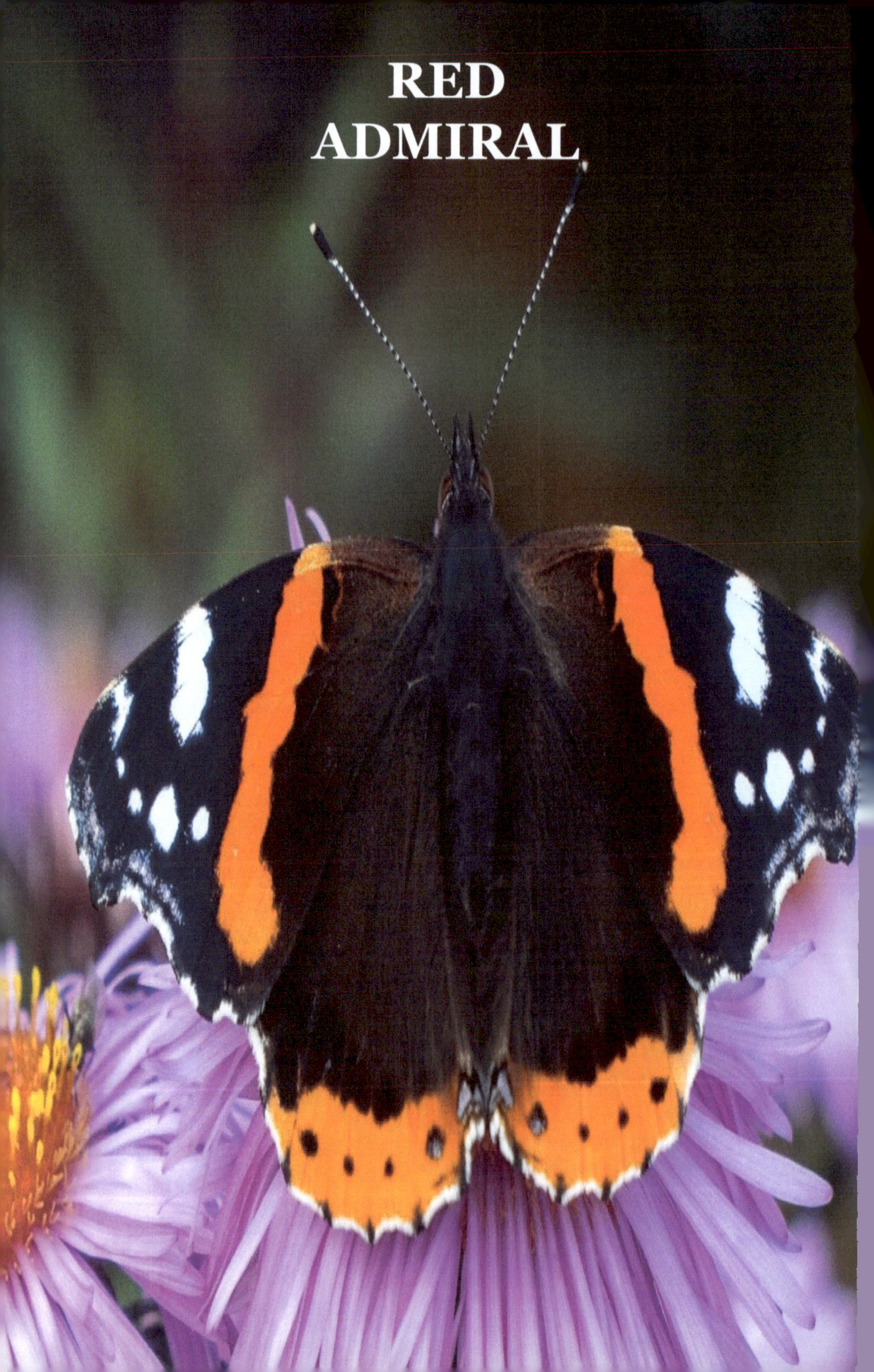
RED
ADMIRAL

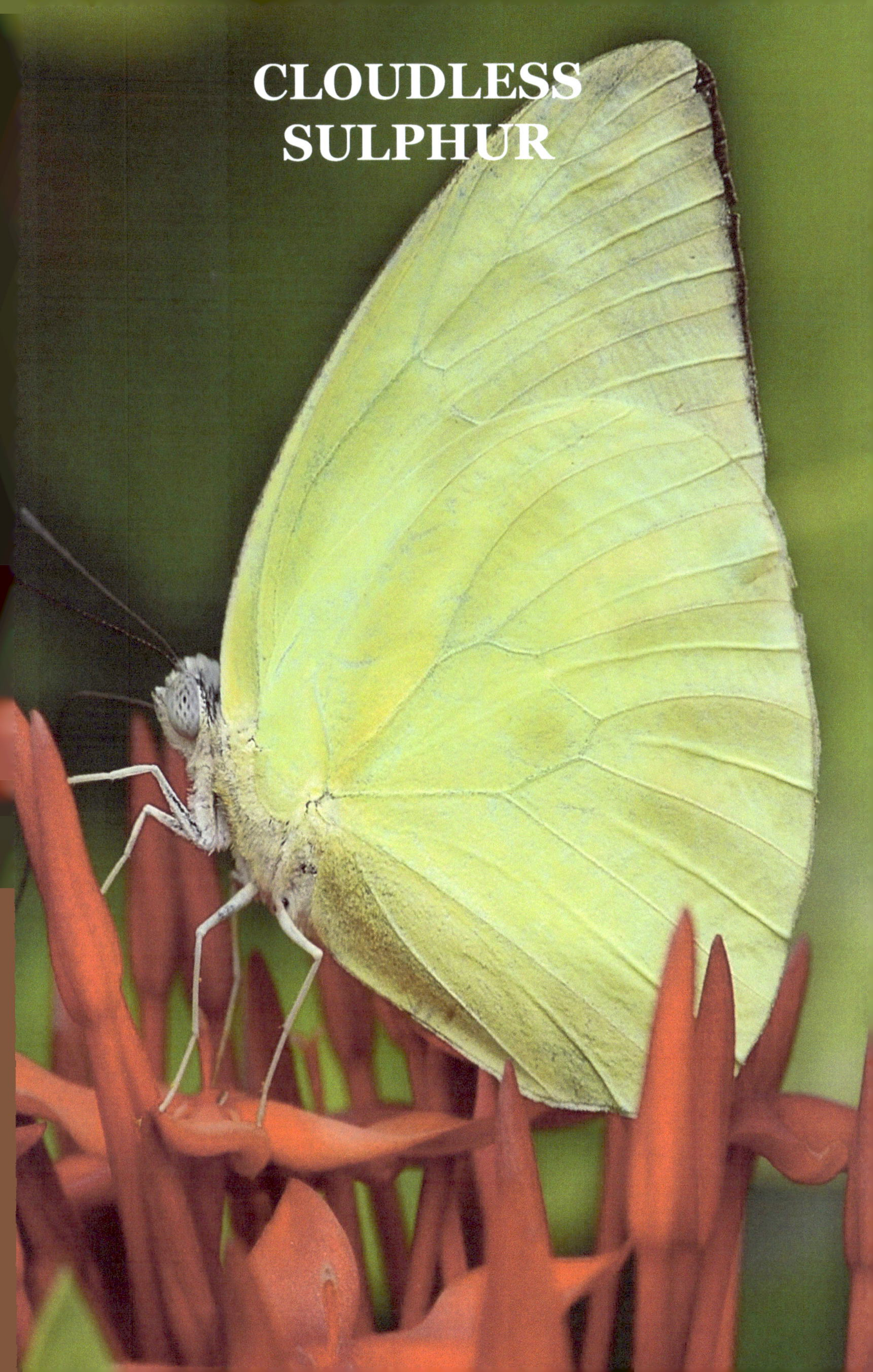
CLOUDLESS
SULPHUR

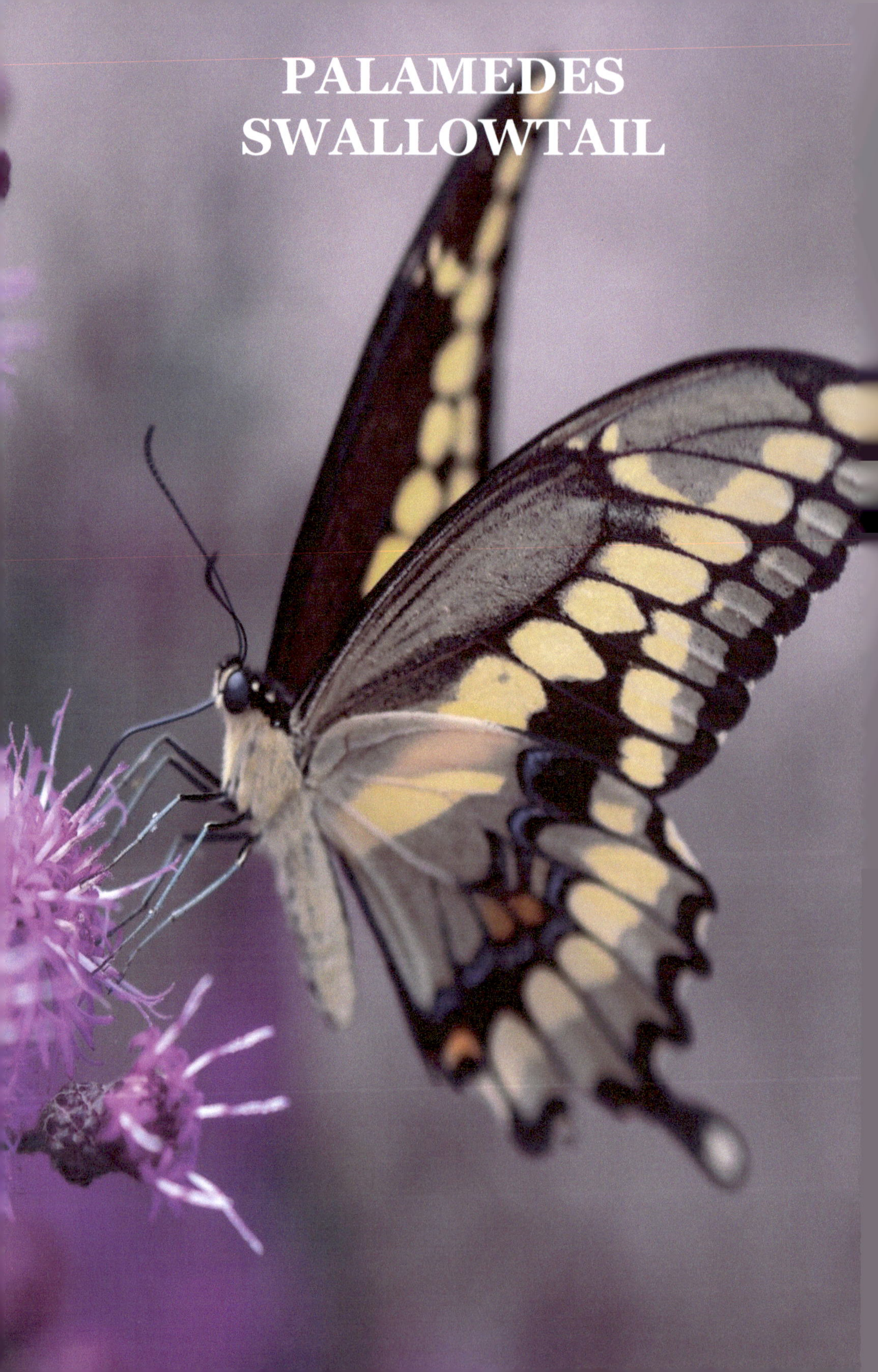
PALAMEDES
SWALLOWTAIL

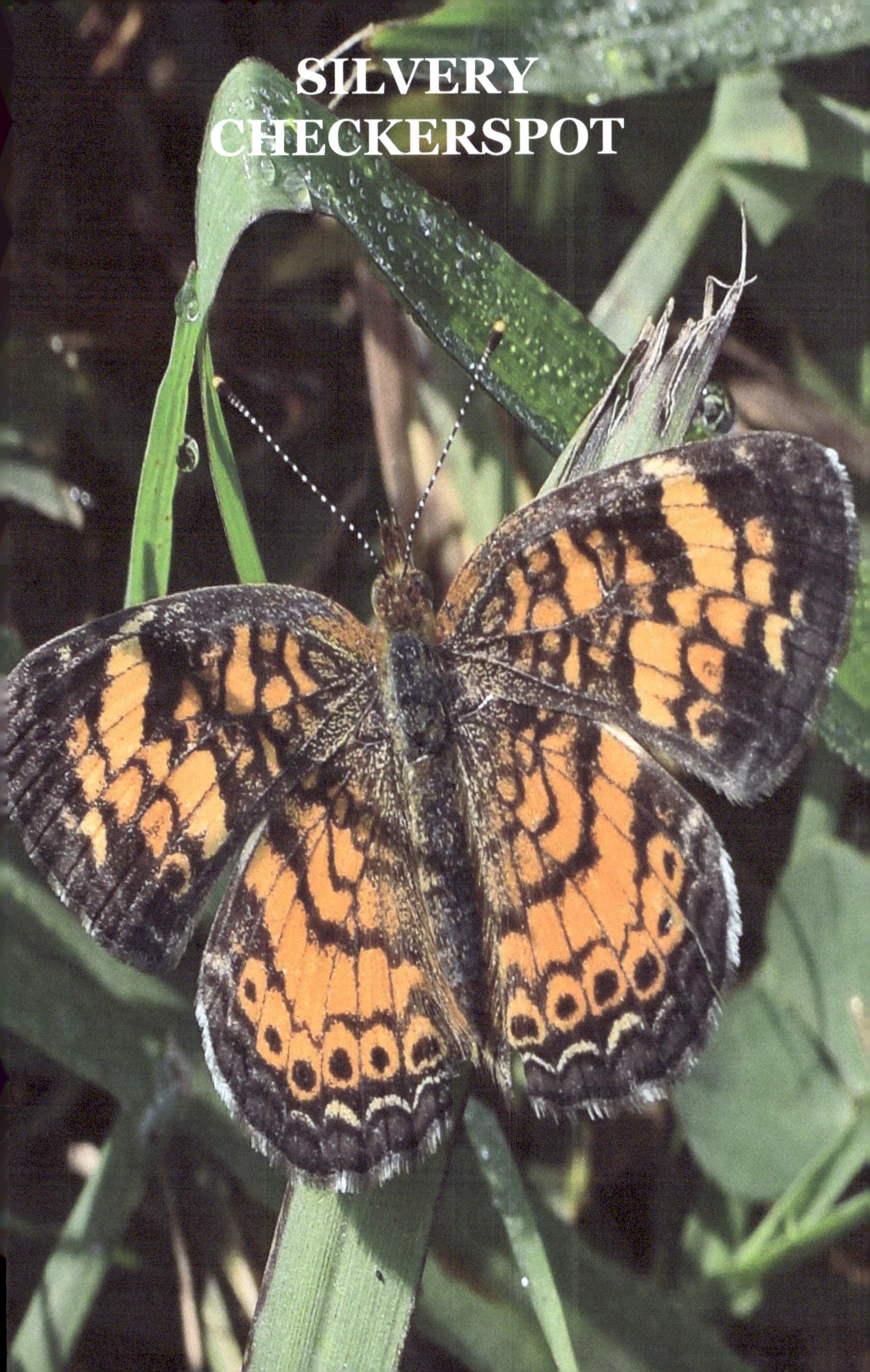
SILVERY
CHECKERSPOT

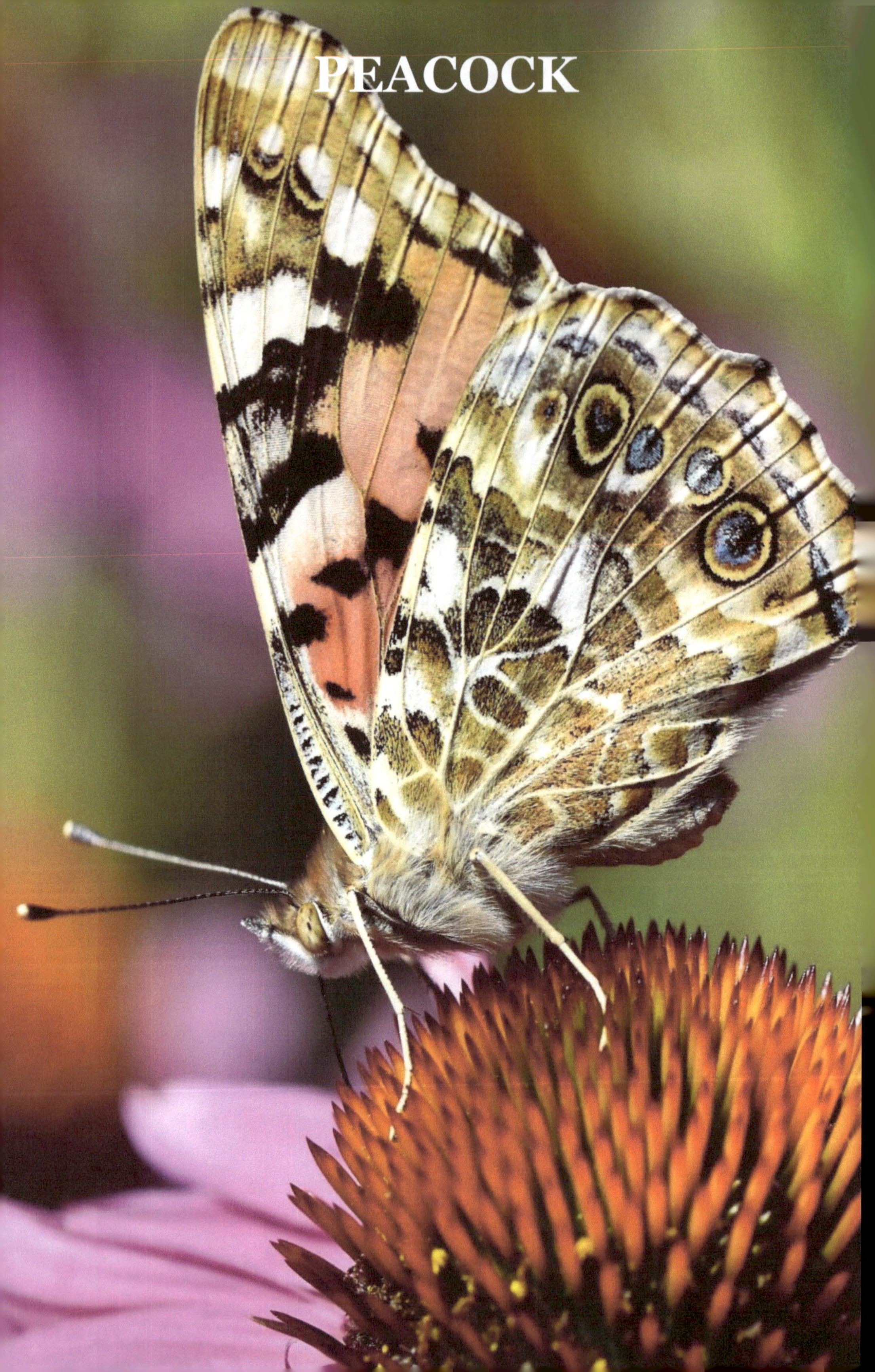
PEACOCK

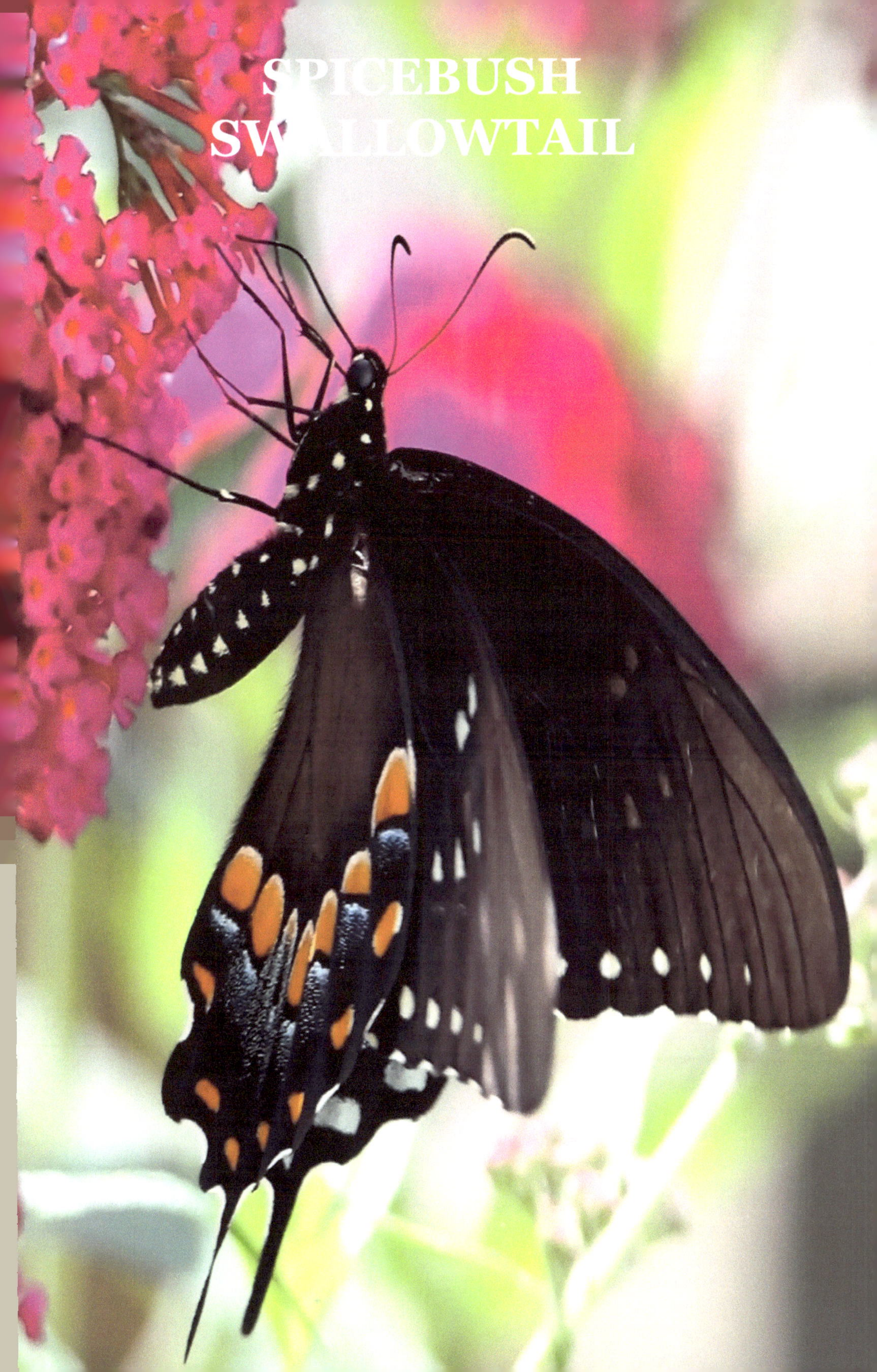
SPICEBUSH
SWALLOWTAIL

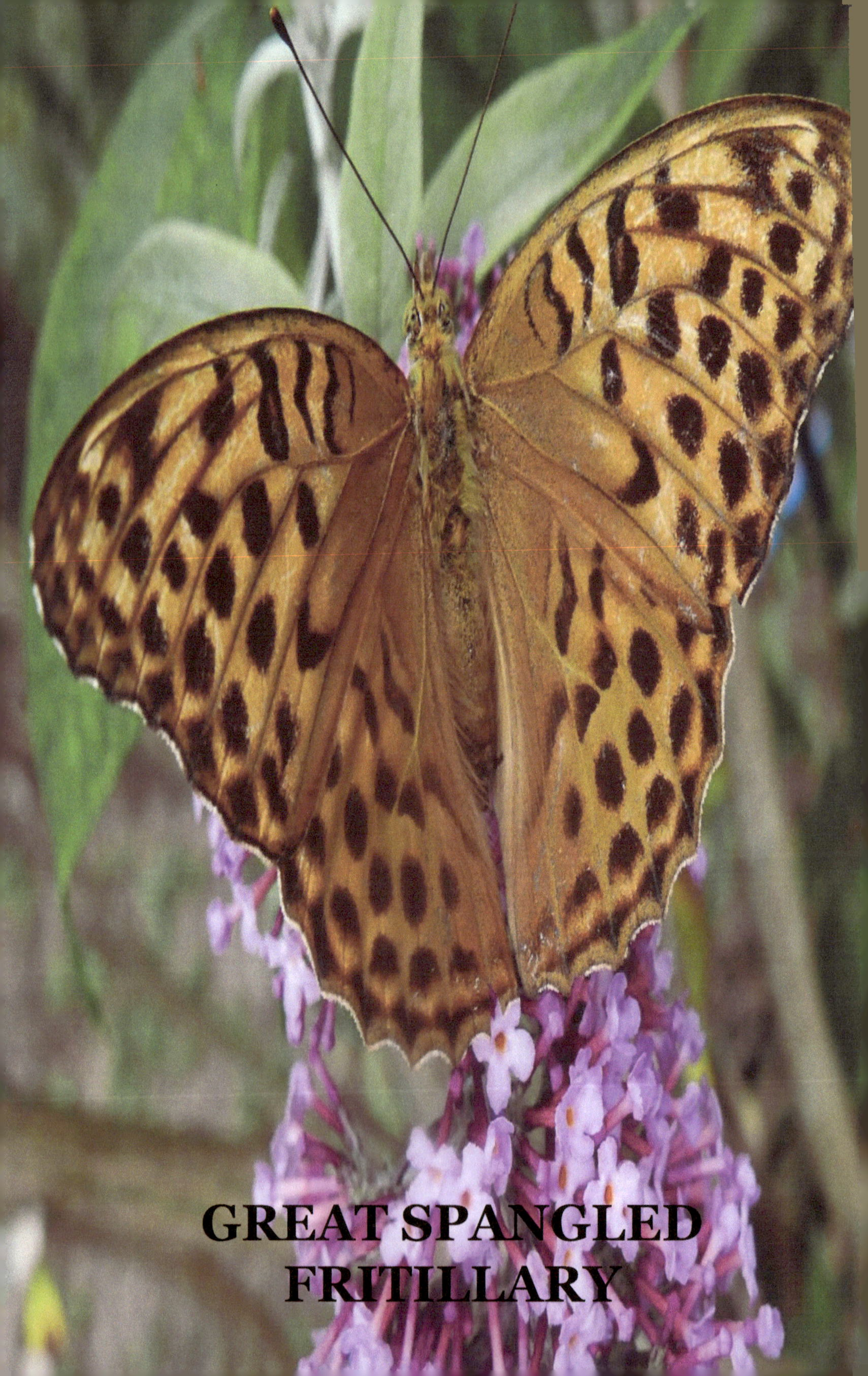

GREAT SPANGLED
FRITILLARY

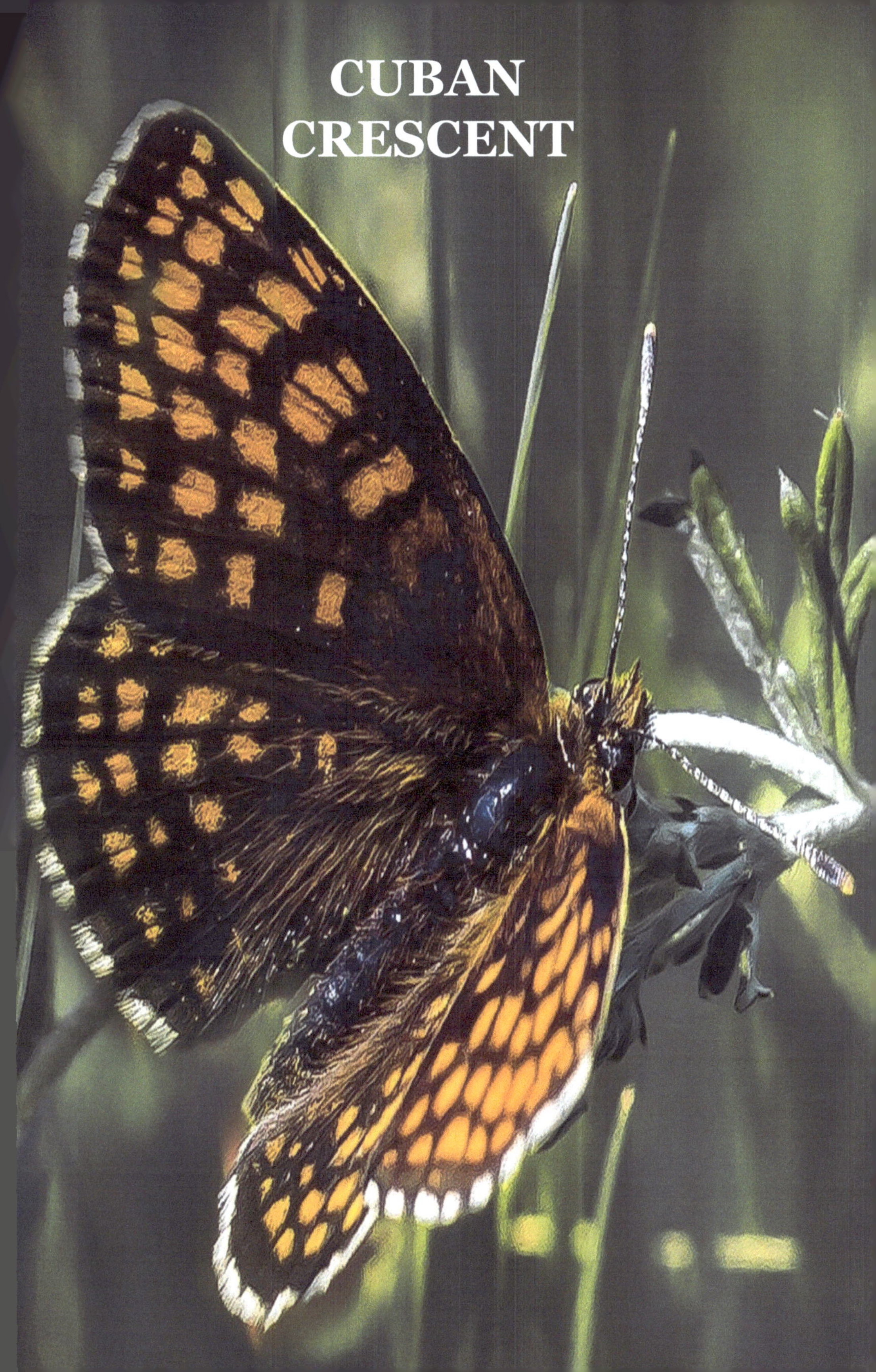

CUBAN
CRESCENT

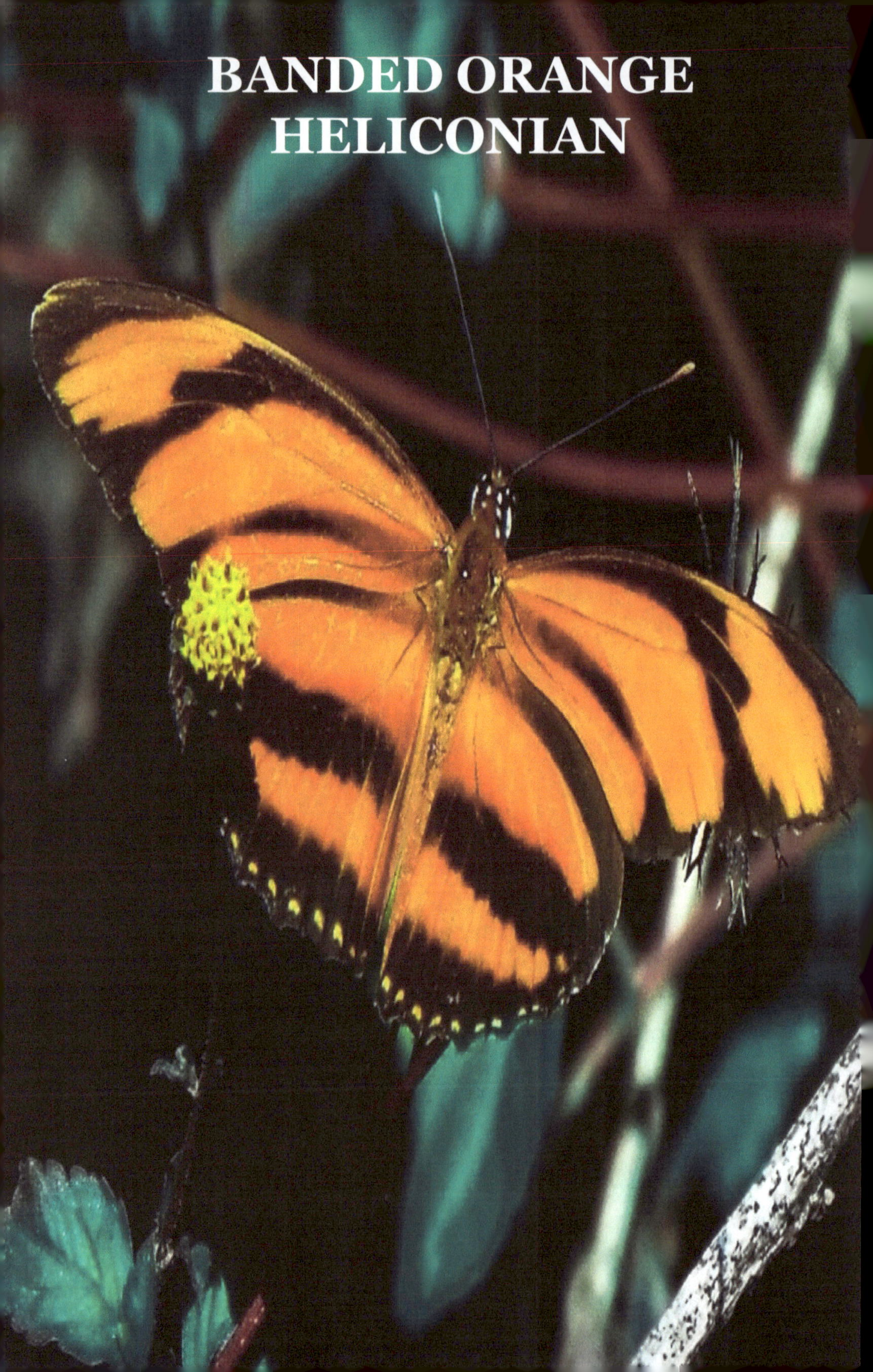

BANDED ORANGE
HELICONIAN

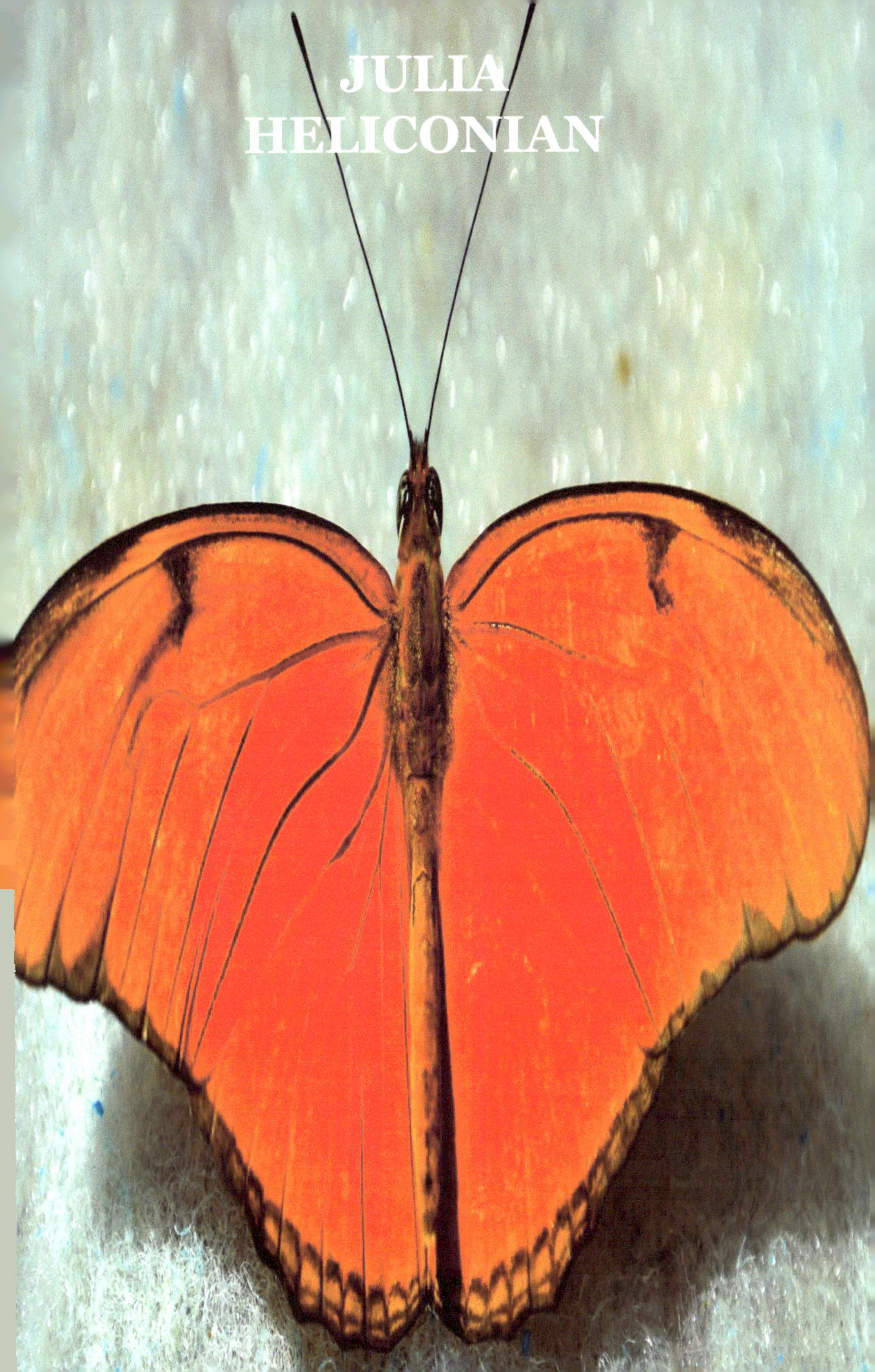
JULIA
HELICONIAN

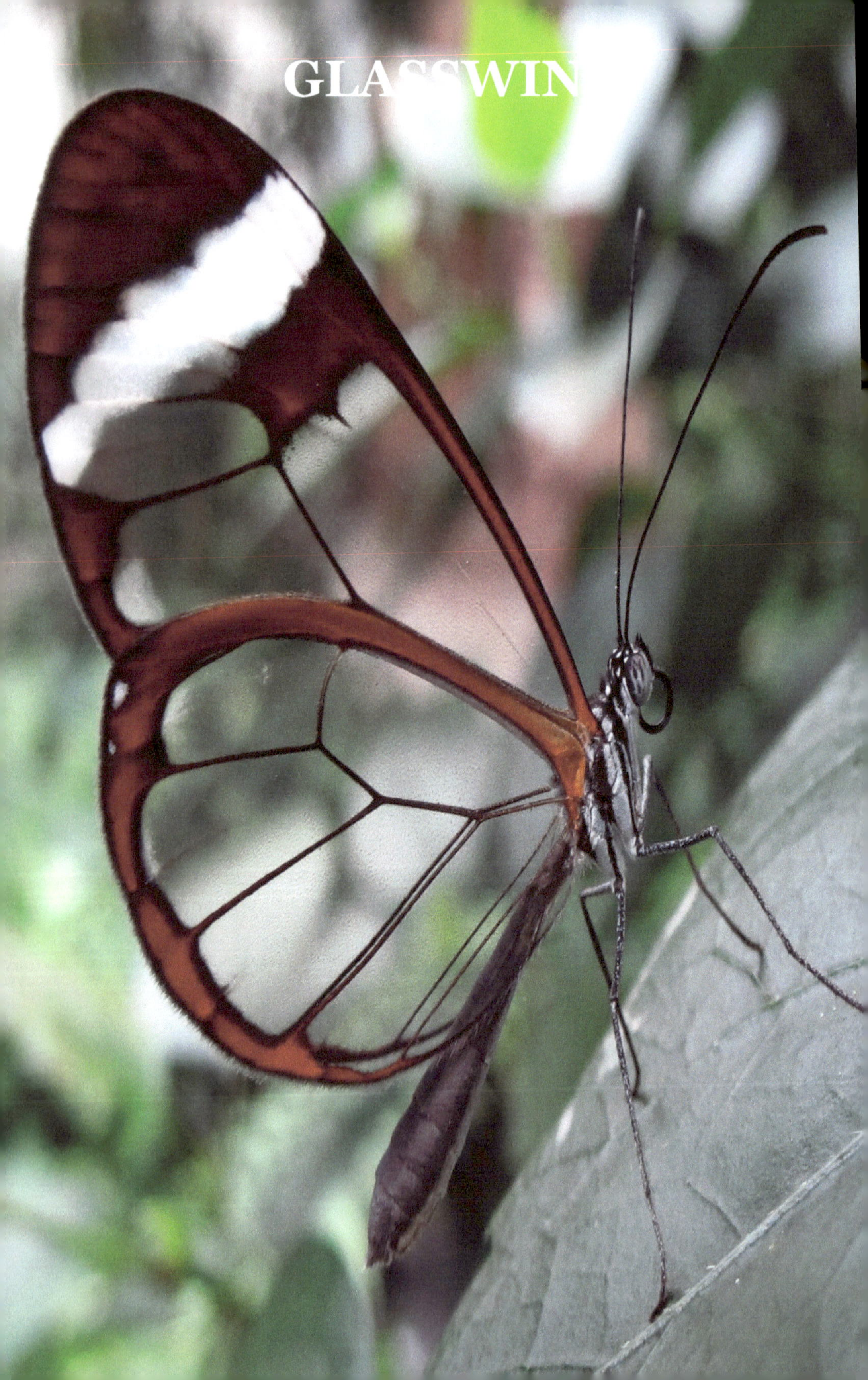
GLASSWIN

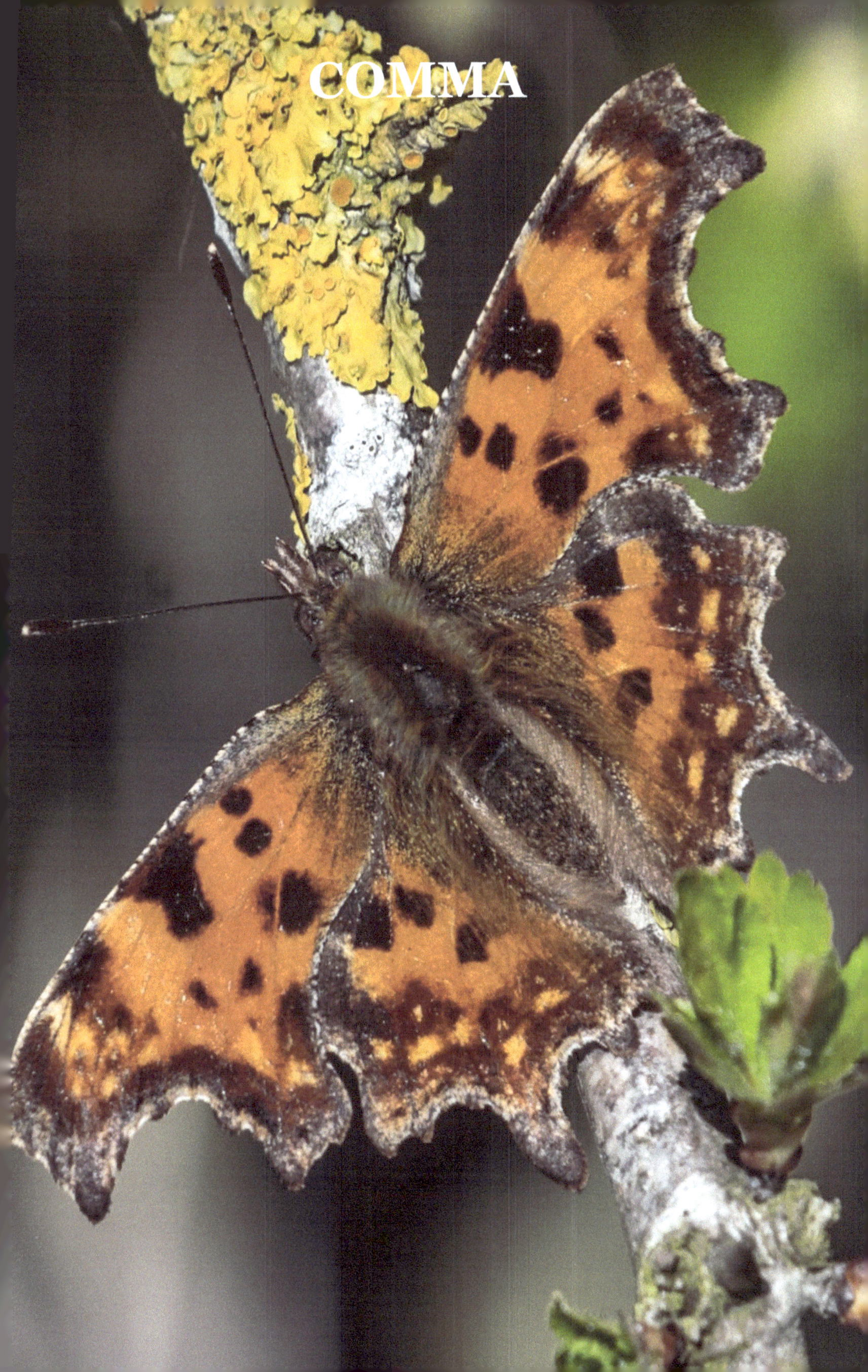
COMMA

NORTHERN CHEQUERED SKIPPER

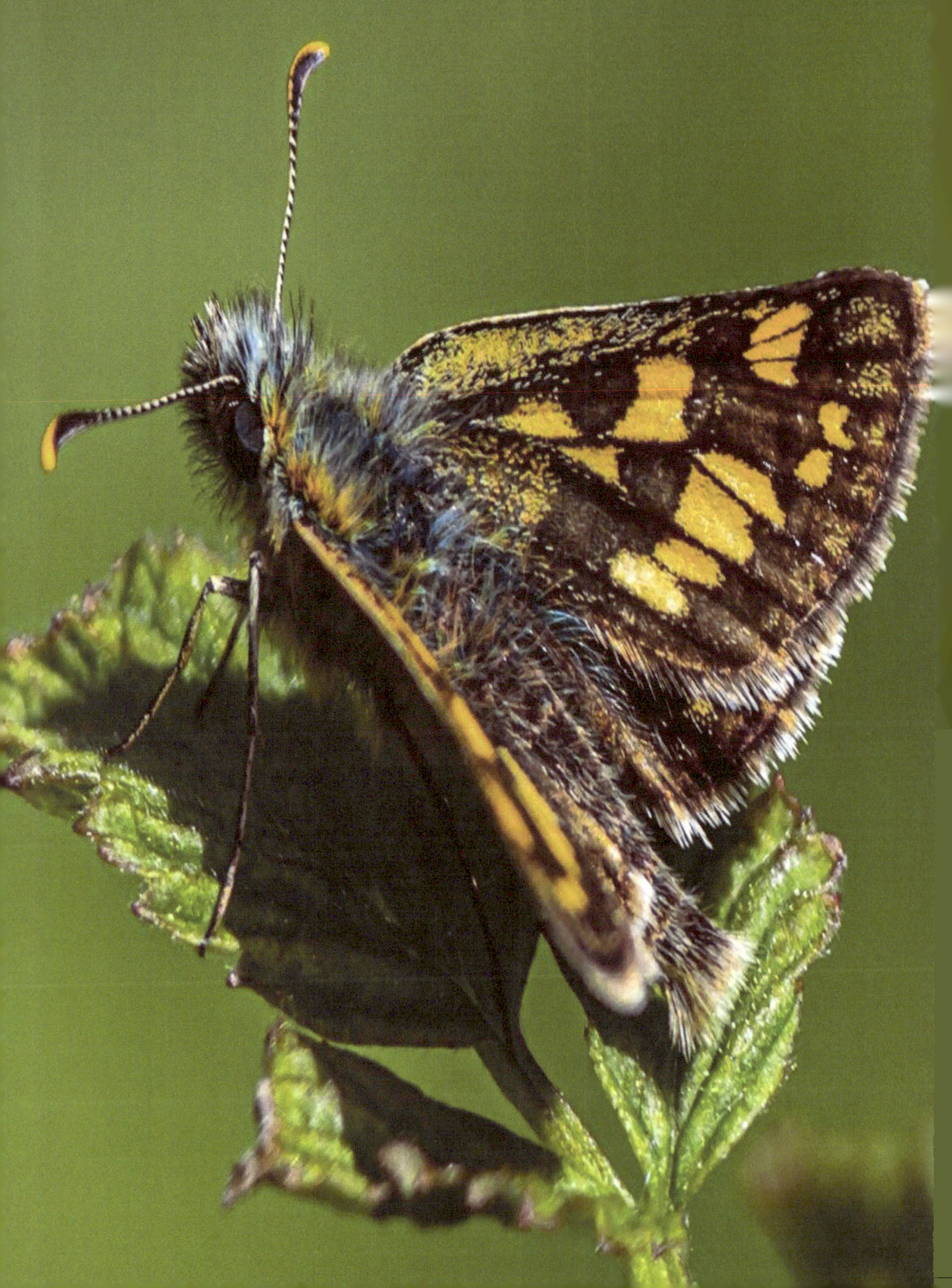

PAINTED LADY

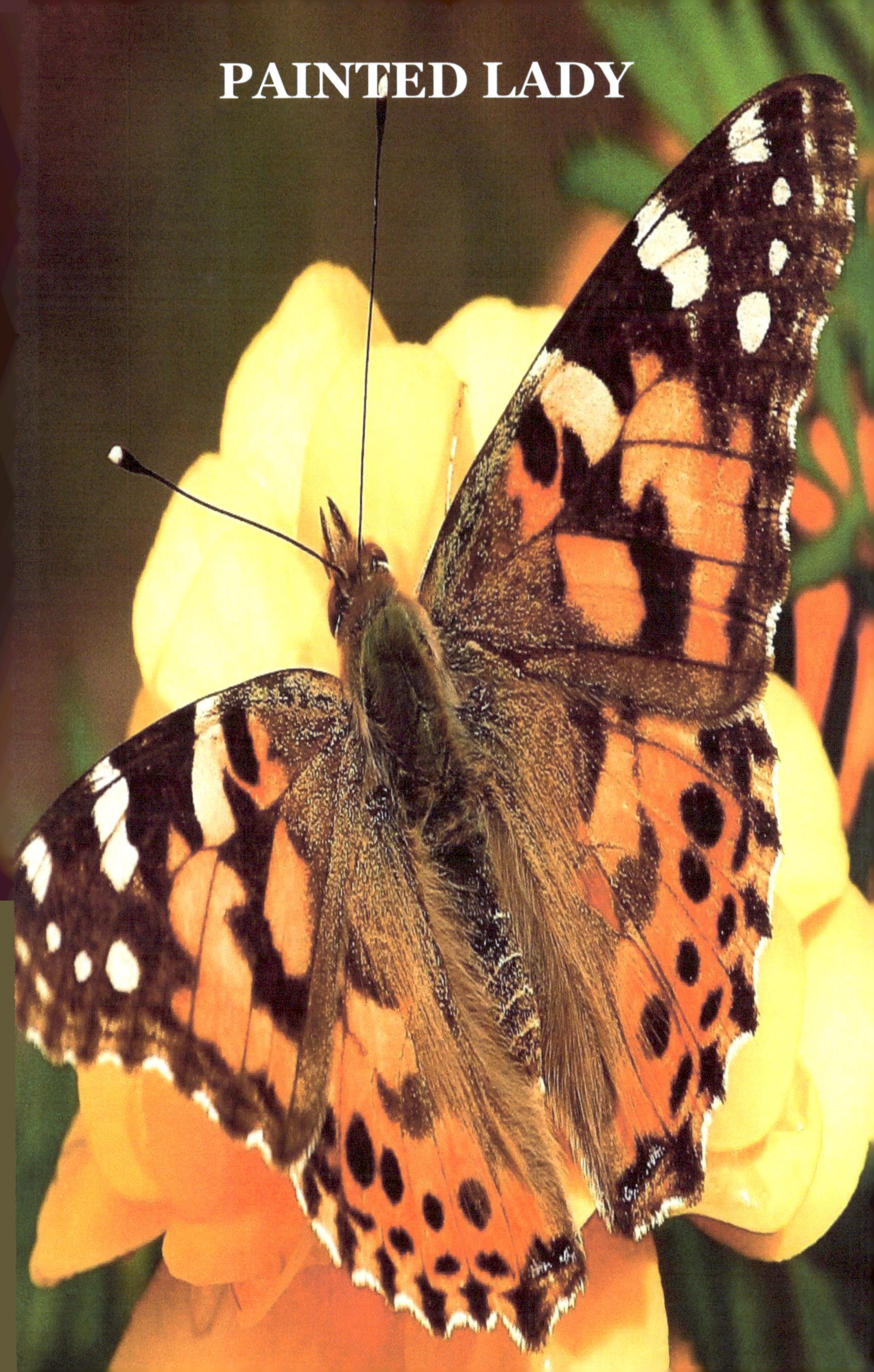

www.ingramcontent.com/pod-product-compliance
Lightning Source LLC
Chambersburg PA
CBHW041807260726
48664CB00035B/1463